CS Checklists

Portable Review for the USMLE Step 2 CS (Clinical Skills Exam)

CS Checklists

Portable Review for the USMLE Step 2 CS (Clinical Skills Exam)

Jennifer K. Rooney, M.D.
Clinical Tutor
St. George's University
Grenada, West Indies

Reviewed by

Patrick Rooney, MD (Hons.), FRCP (Glasgow and Edinburgh), FACP
Department Chair of Clinical Skills
St. George's University
Grenada, West Indies

McGraw-Hill
Medical Publishing Division

New York Chicago San Francisco Lisbon London Madrid Mexico City Milan
New Delhi San Juan Seoul Singapore Sydney Toronto

CS Checklists: Portable Review for the USMLE Step 2 CS (Clinical Skills Exam)

1 2 3 4 5 6 7 8 9 0   DOC/DOC   0 9 8 7 6 5 4

ISBN 0-07-144515-3

This book was set in Electra by PV&M Publishing Solutions.
The editor was Catherine A. Johnson.
The production supervisor was Catherine Saggese.
Project management was provided by Roundhouse Editorial Services.
RR Donnelley was printer and binder.

This book is printed on acid-free paper.

Library of Congress Cataloging-in-Publication Data

Rooney, Jennifer K.
    CS checklists : portable review for the USMLE Step 2 CS (clinical skills exam)
/ [Jennifer K. Rooney].
        p. ; cm.
    ISBN 0-07-144515-3
    1. Physical diagnosis—Examinations, questions, etc.   2. Medical history
taking—Examinations, questions, etc.   3. Diagnosis, Differential—Examinations,
questions, etc.   4. Physicians—Licenses—United States—Examinations—Study
guides.   I. Title: CS checklists.   II. Title: CS.   III. Title.
    [DNLM: 1. Clinical Medicine—Case Reports.   2. Clinical Medicine—
Examinaton Questions. WB 18.2 R777c 2004]
    RC76.R66 2004
    616.07'51'076—dc22

                                                                2004048487

Contents

INTRODUCTION

The Clinical Skills Examination (CSE) is designed to assess the examinee's ability to interact with patients, obtain a history, and perform a physical examination. The ability to communicate the information gathered to colleagues and to the patient is also assessed. The examination is also used to assess proficiency in the English language.

The examination consists of 11 or 12 stations. At each station, the examinee is expected to obtain a history and may have to perform a physical examination. He/she then has to record the findings as well as provide a differential diagnosis and suggested follow-up for the patient. The examinee has approximately 15 minutes in which to obtain the history and perform the physical examination (if required), followed by 10 minutes in which to record the findings, the differential diagnosis, and the follow-up for the patient. The examinee also may be required to provide some feedback and counseling to the patient during the initial 15 minutes. The total duration of the examination is 7–8 hours, including intermittent short breaks and a lunch break.

The examination uses standardized patients who are individuals trained to portray real patients (both by history and by physical examination). The standardized patient responds to questions asked by the examinee and participates in a physical examination. The standardized patients have extensive training and use specific checklists and rating scales to evaluate the examinee. The examination may also be observed by physicians who may assess the examinee's performance and review the final score received by the examinee, ensuring the fairness of the scoring done by the standardized patient.

For many years now, foreign medical students have been required to take the Clinical Skills Assessment Examination (CSA) which is essentially the equivalent of the CSE. The information included in this handbook for the CSE has been gathered from recent foreign graduates who have taken the CSA. Common patient clinical presentations from the examination have been included as well as checklists, differential diagnosis, and follow-up for each patient clinical presentation. The cases which may be presented during the examination are generally representative of the core clerkships of medical schools in the United States. These include internal medicine, pediatrics, surgery, obstetrics/gynecology, psychiatry, and family medicine.

The CSE was launched in the year 2004. The first class required to take the CSE will be the graduating class of 2005. Passing scores in the USMLE step 1 and step 2, along with a passing score in the CSE, will be required for all graduates prior to entering a residency program in the United States. The CSE is incorporated into the USMLE step 2. Candidates may take step 1, step 2, and the CSE in any order, but must pass them prior to taking step 3.

The Step 2 CSE is currently being administered at the following sites: Philadelphia, Atlanta, Los Angeles, Chicago, and Houston. The cost of taking the examination is $975.00 per candidate for US and Canadian medical school students and graduates, and $1200.00 for International Medical Graduates (IMGs).

SECTION 1

Preparation for the CSE

GENERAL INFORMATION

It is recommended that you arrive at the examination center with enough time prior to the start of your examination to sit and relax for a few minutes. The CSE is a lengthy, stressful examination, so take a few minutes to prepare mentally prior to the start of your session.

It is also recommended that you review all of the checklists provided in this handbook as well as to practice patient write-ups prior to the day of the examination.

At each patient station you will wait outside the examination room door and when a buzzer sounds you must enter the room and begin the history/physical examination.

Important Tips

- Dress appropriately (smart professional attire).
- If possible, locate the examination center one day prior to your examination, or earlier on the day of the examination, to avoid any unnecessary stress in trying to find the center at the time of the examination.
- Arrive early for your examination.
- Bring your stethoscope and your white lab coat with you (all other equipment is supplied for you).
- You will be given an orientation/introduction session prior to the start of the examination. Listen carefully to the instructions given to you.
- Be sure to introduce yourself to the patient at each station. Be honest about yourself. If you are a medical student, introduce yourself as such. If you are already a physician, introduce yourself as such.

- Vital signs will be provided to you prior to the start of the patient encounter. Do not repeat them unless it is relevant to the chief complaint; for example, in a patient being seen for a check-up of his/her hypertension.
- *Always* elicit the patient's

  Name

  Age

  Address

  Occupation

  Presenting complaint
- Establish and maintain eye contact with the patient.
- Minimize physical barriers; for example, if there is a desk in the room, have the patient sit at the side of the desk rather than in front of the desk.
- Begin the patient interview using open-ended questions. Allow the patient to respond to the questions without interruption. Avoid multiple questions. Sequence questions appropriately using recap/ summary technique.
- Indicate to the patient that you are paying attention by using non-verbal cues as well as verbal cues. Show empathy to the patient verbally and by posture and body language. Use echoing (repeating the last word or phrase used by the patient) to let the patient know that you are listening and that you are concerned. Use active continuers such as "Go on," "I hear you," and "Tell me more."
- Always acknowledge the patient's feelings and concerns.
- Try to avoid the use of medical or technical terms and always try to ascertain that the patient understands the terms that you are using.
- Prior to the physical examination, explain to the patient what you are planning to do before you actually start the examination.
- Always wash your hands before and after any physical examination of the patient.
- Offer the patient assistance in both getting on and getting off the examination table.
- If the patient is lying on the examination table, be sure to pull out the leg support.

- Never examine the patient through clothing. However, remember to be sensitive to the patient's privacy.
- Rectal, pelvic, genitourinary, female breast, and corneal reflex examinations should not be performed during the examination. If you think that any of these examinations is an important diagnostic step in the case, include it in the follow-up.
- Physical examination checklists in this handbook generally only include components of the physical examination relevant to the patient clinical presentation given. If time permits, other parts of the complete examination may be performed.
- At the end of each patient station explain to the patient your initial diagnostic impressions. You should also inform the patient of any follow-up you would like to have done; for example, lab work, x-rays, and so on. Inform the patient of any changes in lifestyle you would like him/her to attempt and when the most appropriate follow-up visit should take place.
- Remember, your write-up must be legible and should include both positive findings in the history and the physical examination and negative findings. The write-up may be done by hand or typed on a computer.
- The differential diagnoses should be written in order of the most likely diagnosis to the least likely diagnosis.

COMPONENTS OF A COMPLETE HEALTH HISTORY

A complete history should include all of the following:

1. Chief complaint
2. History of the presenting illness
3. Medical history
4. Surgical history
5. Allergies
6. Medications
7. Obstetric/gynecology history
8. Social history
9. Family history
10. Review of systems

Chief Complaint

The chief complaint is what prompted the patient to seek medical care. Try to allow the patient to tell you in his/her own words what the problem is. Open-ended questions are particularly useful for obtaining the chief complaint.

History of the Presenting Illness

This covers the presenting illness from the onset of the symptoms. Allow the patient to relay the events/onset of each symptom as it occurred. After allowing the patient to summarize the history of the illness, direct questions may be useful to obtain further information.

Fully investigate the principal symptoms with descriptions of:

1. Onset
2. Location
3. Character
4. Duration
5. Frequency
6. Severity
7. Aggravating factors
8. Relieving factors
9. Medications taken to relieve symptoms and their effects
10. Associated symptoms
11. The impact on the patient (self, family, occupation)

Medical History

The medical history includes all illnesses that the patient currently has as well as illnesses that they have had in the past which have since resolved, including childhood illnesses. The dates of past illnesses should be established and recorded as well as the dates of onset of any current illnesses. An immunization history should also be included here.

Surgical History

This includes *all* surgeries and the dates of each surgery. Ask specific questions regarding the surgeries if necessary. For example, the reason the patient had the surgery done, whether it was a successful operation, and any complications encountered following the surgery.

Allergies

Inquire about all drug allergies. Also establish the exact reaction that oc-curred when the patient took the specific medication. Inquire about en-vironmental and food allergies.

Medications

Inquire about all medications and their doses that the patient is cur-rently taking. Ask the patient why he/she takes a specific medication, especially if you are unfamiliar with the medication and its uses. Also inquire about medications taken by the patient in the past.

Obstetric/Gynecology History

Inquire about the patient's menstrual cycle and establish the following:

Is it regular?
How often does menstruation occur?
How long does it typically last?
Does the patient have very heavy periods or very painful periods?
When was the last menstrual period?
What age was menarche?
What age was menopause (if relevant)?

Inquire about the patient's obstetric history and establish the following:

How many pregnancies has the patient had?
What was the outcome of each pregnancy?
What was the date of each pregnancy?
What method of birth control does the patient currently use, if any?

Inquire about the patient's sexual history and establish the following:

Is the patient currently sexually active? If so, with how many partners?

Has the patient ever been diagnosed with a sexually transmitted disease?

Female

When was the last pelvic examination done?

When was the last Papanicolaou (Pap) smear?

Has the patient ever had any abnormal Pap smears? If so, what was the treatment or the follow-up required?

Male

Is the patient able to achieve and maintain an erection?

Is ejaculation normal?

What was the date of the last physical examination (including examination of the genitalia)?

Social History

The social history should include the patient's family life, employment situation, and daily habits. A history of alcohol use, cigarette use, and drug use also should be included. Be sure to inquire as to how much, how often, and for what period of time the patient has been using each substance. Other risk behaviors (eg, hang gliding, SCUBA diving) should also be addressed, as well as diet and exercise.

Family History

Inquire about the patient's spouse or partner, parents, siblings, and children. Take note of any medical problems in the family. Pay particular attention to common disorders with an increased contact risk (eg, tuberculosis) or an increased inherited risk (eg, diabetes mellitus or hypertension).

Review of Systems

Following completion of the components of the history, a review of systems can be a useful tool for picking up any symptoms which may not have been mentioned by the patient previously.

The review of systems should consist of an orderly set of questions moving from the head and neck downward. A good model of a systemic inquiry is as follows.

1. General

   How have you been feeling?

   Have you had any recent weight loss or weight gain?

   Have you been feeling tired lately?

2. Head, eyes, ears, nose, throat

   Head

   Have you ever had any problems with or injuries to your head?

   Have you had any headaches?

   Have you experienced any dizziness or lightheadedness?

   Eyes

   Have you ever had any problems with your vision?

   Have you noticed any changes in your vision?

   Have you noticed any blurred or double vision?

   Have you noticed any pain or redness of your eyes?

   Have you noticed any spots or flecks in your visual fields?

   Ears

   Have you ever had any problems with your ears?

   Have you experienced any changes in your hearing?

   Have you noticed any drainage from your ears?

   Have you ever experienced any ringing in your ears?

   Have you ever had any difficulty with your balance?

Nose

Have you ever had any problems with your nose?

Have you had any drainage from your nose?

Do you have any problems or pain from your sinuses?

Do you ever have any nosebleeds?

Do you have any nasal drainage dripping down into your throat?

Throat

Have you ever had any problems with your throat?

Have you had any sore throats?

Do you ever experience bleeding gums?

When was your last visit to your dentist?

Do you have artificial dentition?

3. Neck

Have you ever had any problems with your neck?

Have you noticed any lumps?

Have you had any stiffness of your neck?

Have you noticed any difficulty swallowing?

4. Cardiovascular

Have you ever had any problems with your heart?

Do you ever experience chest pain?

Do you ever feel palpitations?

Do you ever feel short of breath?

Do you ever wake up during the night feeling short of breath?

Do you ever notice any swelling of your legs?

5. Respiratory

Have you ever had any problems with your breathing?

Are you ever short of breath? If so, when?

Do you have a cough? If so, is the cough productive?

Do you ever have any chest pain?

6. Breast

    Have you ever had any problems with your breasts?

    Do you do self–breast examinations? How often?

    Do you ever have painful breasts?

    Have you ever noticed any lumps?

    Do you have any nipple discharge?

7. Gastrointestinal

    Have you ever had any problems with your stomach or bowels?

    How is your appetite?

    Have you noticed any change in your appetite?

    Do you have any difficulty swallowing?

    Do you ever experience heartburn?

    Do you ever experience abdominal pain?

    Have you ever vomited blood?

    Are your bowel movements regular?

    Have you ever noticed any blood in your stool?

8. Urinary

    Have you ever had any problems with urination?

    Do you have any pain during urination?

    Do you notice any increased frequency of urination?

    Do you have any blood in your urine?

    Male

    Is your urinary stream normal?

    Do you notice any reduced force of the urinary stream?

    Do you ever have any difficulty urinating (hesitancy)?

    Do you ever have any dribbling (incontinence)?

9. Musculoskeletal

    Have you ever had any problems with your bones or joints?

    Do you have any joint stiffness?

    Do you ever have any pain, swelling, or redness of any joints?

    Do you have any limitation of activity due to muscle or joint pain?

10. Neurological

> Have you ever had any neurologic problems?
>
> Do you ever experience dizziness?
>
> Have you ever fainted?
>
> Have you ever experienced any numbness or paralysis? If so, where?
>
> Do you have any weakness of your arms or legs?

11. Hematologic

> Have you ever had any bleeding problems?
>
> Do you ever experience easy bruising?
>
> Have you ever had a blood transfusion for any reason?

12. Psychiatric

> Have you ever had any psychiatric illnesses?
>
> Have you ever had any problems with depression?
>
> Have you ever had any problems with anxiety?
>
> Have you ever had any suicidal thoughts (if yes to any of the above)?

COMPONENTS OF A COMPLETE PHYSICAL EXAMINATION

General Assessment

Observe the patient as he/she enters the room. Observe the patient's gait, height, sexual development, and posture. Observe the patient's clothing and hygiene. Be aware of any odors on the patient's breath or body.

Vital Signs

As the name indicates, these are a vital component of any examination.

Temperature

Pulse

    Rate

    Rhythm

    Volume

    Character

    Condition of the vessel wall

    Comparison of both radial arteries

    Assess for radio-femoral delay

Blood Pressure

    Measure in three positions

        Sitting

        Standing

        Supine

Measure the blood pressure by palpation of the radial artery in any new patient before auscultation over the brachial artery

Compare the blood pressure in both arms in one of the three positions

Respirations
Rate
Rhythm
Regularity
Thoracic or abdominal

Skin

When examining any mucosal surface or any area of potentially infected or broken skin *remember to use gloves.*

Inspect for lesions, scars, and rashes

Inspect the nails and the hair

Head and Neck

Examine and Palpate the Head
Size, shape, contour, deformities, suture lines
Facial expression and symmetry
Abnormal movements of the face

Examine the Scalp
Hair distribution and texture
Swellings
Nits and lice

Examine the Oral Cavity
   Lips
   Buccal mucosa
   Gums and teeth
   Roof of the mouth
   Soft palate
   Uvula
   Pharynx
   Tonsils
   Tongue
   Floor of the mouth
   Salivary glands

Examine and Palpate the Neck
   Anatomical landmarks
   Lymph nodes
   Position of the trachea

Thyroid Gland (Isthmus and Lateral Lobes)
   Inspect (directly and on swallowing)
   Palpate (directly and on swallowing)
   Auscultate

Ears, Nose, and Sinuses

Ears

Inspect the external ears for deformities, discharge, symmetry, lesions, inflammation

Palpate

Tragus

Auricle

Mastoid process

Inspect the external canal with an ear speculum

Inspect the tympanic membrane for color, cone of light, handle of malleus, incus, perforations, and retractions

Perform the whisper test

Perform Weber's test

Perform Rinne's test

Nose and Sinuses

Inspect the nostrils for patency, asymmetry, deformities, color, and discharge

Inspect the nasal mucosa bilaterally, using the nasal speculum, for color, discharge, bleeding, and nasal polyps

Inspect the nasal septum for deviation or perforation

Palpate the frontal and maxillary sinuses

Transilluminate the frontal and the maxillary sinuses

Eyes

Examine the eyebrows for hair distribution and rashes

Examine the eyes for alignment

Examine the eyelids for swellings, lesions, ptosis, or lid retraction

Check the visual acuity and the peripheral visual fields with and without any corrective lenses used by the patient

Examine the conjunctiva for color, inflammation, or lesions

Examine the lacrimal punctae and lacrimal sac for obstruction, discharge, or inflammation

Examine the anterior chamber for clarity. Note any abnormal contents (eg, blood, pus)

Examine the extraocular muscles

Examine the iris for color, inflammation, arcus, or other abnormalities

Note any surgical scars

Examine the pupils for equality, shape, lens opacities, and reflexes

Using the ophthalmoscope, observe the retina

Cardiovascular System

Examine the face for pallor or cyanosis

Examine the hands for clubbing, cyanosis, or signs of bacterial endocarditis

Examine the lower extremities bilaterally for pitting edema

Examine the neck

> Examine the jugular venous pulse wave pattern
>
> Measure the jugular venous pressure and assess for any sustained hepatojugular reflux
>
> Assess the carotid arteries for bruits

Inspect the precordium for shape, symmetry, apical beat, and pulsations

Note any surgical scars

Palpate for tenderness

Palpate the cardiac areas as follows:

> Aortic
>
> Pulmonic
>
> Erb's point
>
> Tricuspid
>
> Apex (mitral)

Locate the apex and note the site, size, and character of the apical beat

Palpate for pulsations and thrills in other cardiac areas including the epigastrium

Look for a right ventricular heave

Percuss the right and left borders of the heart

Auscultate all areas with both the bell and the diaphragm

Respiratory System

Examine the head, neck, and chest for the use of accessory muscles of respiration

Examine the hands and face for cyanosis and for the presence of finger clubbing

Listen for hoarseness of the voice, wheezing, and coughing

Inspect the nose for lesions

Examine the throat for lesions

Palpate the trachea for deviation

Inspect the anterior chest for symmetry and deformities

Palpate the chest for tenderness, tactile vocal fremitus, and chest excursion

Percuss symmetrical areas of the chest starting from the apex

Auscultate starting from the apices (during percussion and auscultation always compare the same areas on each side)

Assess the character of the breath sounds

Assess vocal resonance

Assess for egophony

Assess for whispering pectoriloquy

Repeat all examinations on the posterior chest

Assess the level and excursion of the diaphragm at the posterior chest by palpation and percussion

Abdomen

Examine the mouth for signs of vitamin deficiencies

Examine the mouth for presence and status of teeth and the presence of any dental caries

Examine the hands and the arms for signs of hepatic failure (palmar erythema, leukonychia, asterixis)

Examine the conjunctiva and the mucous membranes for signs of jaundice

Examine the anterior chest for spider angiomas and gynecomastia

Expose the abdomen from the mid chest to the thighs

Inspect the abdomen for shape, size, color, symmetry, striae, hair distribution, scars, dilated venous patterns (caput medusae or obstruction of the inferior vena cava), visible peristalsis, visible pulsations, and fetal movements (if relevant)

Auscultate the abdomen for bowel sounds, bruits over the renal arteries, and friction rubs over the spleen and the liver

Palpate the abdomen starting away from any area of pain or tenderness

  Light palpation

  Deep palpation (check for any masses or areas of tenderness)

  Assess the lower border of the liver

  Assess the tip of the spleen (patient lying flat and also on his/her right side)

  Palpate the kidneys

  Percuss the upper and the lower borders of the liver, the spleen, and the bladder

Evaluate for a fluid wave and shifting dullness

If appendicitis is suspected, check for

  Rebound tenderness

  Rovsing's sign

  Psoas sign

  Obturator sign

If cholecystitis is suspected, check for

> Murphy's sign
>
> Boas' sign

In any patient in whom you suspect significant abdominal pathology do a digital rectal examination. (In the CSE, state to the patient that you wish to do this but will not do so during this examination.)

Musculoskeletal System

Examine individual groups of joints

Compare symmetrical joints

Inspect each joint for swelling, redness, deformities, condition of the surrounding tissues, and active range of motion

Palpate each joint for tenderness, warmth, and crepitus. If the active range of motion is impaired, check the passive range of motion

Examine the axial skeleton (temporomandibular joints; cervical, dorsal, and lumbar spine) in the same manner

Perform additional tests for the knee joint

> Bulge sign
>
> Ballottement
>
> Drawer sign and assessment of collateral ligaments
>
> McMurray's test

Examine for sciatic nerve compression—straight leg raising test

Examine for hip flexion contractures—Thomas' test

Examine for median nerve compression—Phalen's test and Tinel's sign

Peripheral Vascular System

Inspect the upper and lower extremities for size and symmetry

Examine the nails, hair, and skin

Observe any ulcers or gangrene (always remember to inspect the soles of the feet, especially in diabetic patients)

Palpate temperature in both the upper and the lower extremities, comparing both limbs

Palpate pulses

Dorsalis pedis

Posterior tibial

Popliteal

Femoral

Radial

Ulnar

Brachial

Perform Allen's test

Perform Buerger's test

If you suspect that the patient has venous problems, assess for edema and measure the size of the calf. Perform the Trendelenberg test, the manual compression test, the Pratt's test, and the Homan's test.

Central Nervous System

Evaluate mental status (a mini mental state examination can be used)

Orientation to person, place, and time

Level of consciousness

Short-term memory

Long-term memory

Abstract or concrete thinking

Observe the patient's gait and speech

Examine all cranial nerves (I–XII)

CN I

Test nostrils for patency

Ask patient to identify common aromatic substances

CN II

Test visual acuity

Test pupillary reflexes (direct and consensual)

Test accommodation reflexes

CN III, IV, VI

Assess pupillary reactions to light

Assess corneal reflection

Perform H test for extraocular muscles

CN V

Assess pain, touch, and fine touch in each division of the nerve

Elicit corneal reflex

Assess strength of muscles of mastication

CN VII

Ask patient to wrinkle forehead, close eyes, smile, and blow out cheeks

CN VIII

Perform whisper, Weber, and Rinne tests

CN IX, X

Assess movements of soft palate

Assess gag reflex

CN XI

Assess strength of trapezius and sternocleidomastoid muscles

CN XII

Ask patient to protrude tongue (assess for fasciculations, atrophy, and deviations)

Sensory System

Check for pain, crude touch, and fine touch in all parts of the body
Check sensations carried by the dorsal columns
    Romberg's test
    Proprioception at fingers and toes
    Vibratory sense
Check sensations of the parietal cortex
    Stereognosis
    Graphesthesia
    2-point discrimination
    Point localization
    Extinction

Motor System

Inspect the motor system for atrophy, fasciculations, and involuntary
    movements
Palpate all limbs for muscle tone
Check all major muscle groups for power
Check all reflexes
    Abdominal
    Plantar
    Biceps
    Triceps
    Brachioradialis
    Knee
    Ankle

Cerebellum

Ask the patient to walk in a straight line, heel to toe
Ask the patient to walk in a straight line on his/her heels
Ask the patient to walk in a straight line on his/her toes
Ask the patient to perform the finger–nose test
Ask the patient to perform the knee–heel–shin test
Check for dysdiadochokinesia (in both hands and feet)

COMPLETE WRITE-UP

Remember: The write-up should be legible. No points will be given if the examiners are unable to read what you have written.

Areas that will be evaluated include:

1. Organization. Is the write-up easy to interpret? Does the content flow smoothly from one area to the next?
2. Accuracy. Does the write-up reflect the data obtained during the patient encounter? Is the write-up complete?
3. Analysis. Are the differential diagnoses appropriate? Is there information elsewhere in the write-up to support each differential diagnosis?
4. Management. Is the follow-up appropriate? Does the follow-up correspond to the differential diagnosis listed?
5. Clarity. Is the note legible? Is the use of language appropriate?

Example: Ectopic Pregnancy

Chief Complaint

Abdominal pain for the past 24 hours

History of Presenting Illness

The patient is a 23-year-old female complaining of abdominal pain for the past 24 hours. She describes the pain as dull and aching and located in the pelvic area. The pain does not radiate. The patient rates the pain a 7 on a scale of 1–10, with 10 being the worst. The pain has been worsening over the past 24 hours since the onset. She has had no nausea, vomiting, or diarrhea. Patient denies fever. Her last menstrual period was approximately 5 weeks ago. Patient reports that her periods are often irregular but never as late as this. She is sexually active with one partner, her husband, and denies vaginal discharge. She and her husband use condoms as a method of birth control. She has no dysuria/frequency or urgency. The patient has been healthy in the past and denies ever having experienced this pain before. Her appetite has been poor since the onset of the pain. She has not taken any medications to try to relieve the pain. The patient denies constipation and reports that her last bowel movement was 1 day ago.

Medical History

Urinary tract infection, 1 year ago

Surgical History

Tonsillectomy, age 6

Medications

Tylenol as needed

Social History

Patient lives with her husband and their 2-year-old child (female). Both are in good health

There are no pets at home

The patient is employed as a bank teller

She smokes approximately ½ a pack of cigarettes per day

She denies the use of alcohol

Family History

Patient's mother and father are alive

Her mother and her maternal grandmother suffer from hypertension

Her maternal grandfather suffered from asthma

She has 3 male siblings who are all healthy

Obstetric/Gynecologic History

Menstrual periods approximately every 28 days

She has no dysmenorrhea/menorrhagia or metrorrhagia

She has had 1 pregnancy 2 years ago, resulting in the vaginal delivery of a healthy female infant

Her last menstrual period was approximately 5 weeks ago

Her last Pap smear was 9 months ago. She has no history of abnormal Pap smears

She is sexually active with one partner and they use condoms

She has no history of sexually transmitted diseases

Physical Examination (Focused Examination)

General: 23-year-old Caucasian female in mild distress

Vitals

Temperature: 98.1°F

Pulse: 94

Blood pressure: 134/86

Respirations: 14

Eyes: No conjunctival pallor noted

Mouth

No cracks/fissures noted

Mucous membranes moist

No pallor

No dental caries noted

Abdomen

No ecchymosis visible

No visible masses

No striae noted

No visible peristalsis

Bowel sounds present in all quadrants

No bruits heard

No friction rubs over the spleen or liver

Mild tenderness in the left lower quadrant to mild palpation

Marked tenderness in the left lower quadrant to deep palpation

No hepatosplenomegaly

No costovertebral angle (CVA) tenderness

No shifting dullness

No rebound tenderness

Rovsing's sign negative

Psoas sign negative

Obturator sign negative

Differential Diagnosis

1. Ectopic pregnancy
2. Ruptured ovarian cyst
3. Appendicitis
4. Ovarian torsion
5. Urinary tract infection

Follow-Up

1. Digital rectal examination (DRE)
2. Beta human chorionic gonadotrophin (β-HCG)
3. Urinalysis (U/A)
4. Complete blood count (CBC)
5. Abdominal ultrasound

ACCEPTABLE ABBREVIATIONS

Note: This is not a complete list of acceptable abbreviations that may be used during the examination but rather a representative sample of common abbreviations that may be used on a patient note. If you are uncertain about the correct abbreviation on exam day, write it out.

Vital Signs

BP	Blood pressure
HR	Heart rate
R	Respirations
T	Temperature
JVP	Jugular venous pulse or pressure

Laboratory Tests and Follow-Up

ABG	Arterial blood gas
β-HCG	Beta human chorionic gonadotrophin
BUN	Blood urea nitrogen
CABG	Coronary artery bypass grafting
CBC	Complete blood count
CK level	Creatinine phosphokinase level
CK-MB	Creatine kinase (myocardial component)
CPR	Cardiopulmonary resuscitation
CT	Computerized tomography
CVP	Central venous pressure
CXR	Chest x-ray
DRE	Digital rectal examination

ECG	Electrocardiogram
EcHO	Echocardiogram
EEG	Electroencephalogram
EGD	Esophagogastroduodenoscopy
EMG	Electromyography
ERCP	Endoscopic retrograde cholangiopancreatography
ESR	Erythrocyte sedimentation rate
Free T_3	Free triiodothyroxine
Free T_4	Free thyroxine
HgA1C	Glycosylated hemoglobin level
IM	Intramuscular
IV	Intravenous
LFT	Liver function test
LP	Lumbar puncture
MRI	Magnetic resonance imaging
PFT	Pulmonary function test
PPD	Purified protein derivative (tuberculin skin test)
PT	Prothrombin time
PTT	Partial prothrombin time
RBC	Red blood cells
RF	Rheumatoid factor
TPA	Tissue plasminogen activator
TSH	Thyroid stimulating hormone
U/A	Urinalysis
VDRL	Venereal Disease Research Laboratory
WBC	White blood cells

Units of Measure

C	Centigrade
cm	Centimeter
F	Fahrenheit
g	Gram
hr	Hour
kg	Kilogram
m	Meter
μg	Microgram
mg	Milligram
min	Minute
oz	Ounces
lbs	Pounds

Other

AIDS	Acquired immunodeficiency syndrome
CCU	Cardiac care unit
CHF	Congestive heart failure
COPD	Chronic obstructive pulmonary disease
CVA	Cerebrovascular accident
DM	Diabetes mellitus
DTR	Deep tendon reflexes
ENT	Ear, nose, and throat
EOM	Extraocular muscles
ETOH	Alcohol
Ext	Extremities
FH	Family history
GI	Gastrointestinal

GU	Genitourinary
HEENT	Head, ears, eyes, nose, and throat
HIV	Human immunodeficiency virus
HTN	Hypertension
JVD	Jugular venous distention
KUB	Kidney, ureter, and bladder
LMP	Last menstrual period
MVA	Motor vehicle accident
NIDDM	Noninsulin-dependent diabetes mellitus
NKA	No known allergies
NKDA	No known drug allergies
NL	Normal limits
NSAID	Nonsteriodal anti-inflammatory drug
NSR	Normal sinus rhythm
PA	Posteroanterior
PERRLA	Pupils equal, round, reactive to light and accommodation
Po	Per os (orally)
TIA	Transient ischemic attack
URI	Upper respiratory infection
WNL	Within normal limits
yo	year-old

Patient Clinical Presentations and Checklists

AIDS

A 25-year-old male is seen in the outpatient clinic complaining of diarrhea. He states that the diarrhea started approximately 2 weeks ago and is so severe that it is interfering with his job. He has been having diarrhea 8–10 a day. He complains of some mild abdominal discomfort associated with the diarrhea. There is no blood or mucus in the stool. His appetite has been poor and he has been having some difficulty sleeping. When questioned about his medical history he tells the physician that he is HIV positive. He was first tested 3 years ago when he had an outbreak of shingles. He has had 2 episodes of pneumonia; however, he cannot remember the name of the organism involved. He is currently taking retrovir, combivir, and bactrim.

Patient History Checklist

- ☐ Patient's name
- ☐ Patient's age
- ☐ Patient's address
- ☐ Patient's occupation
- ☐ Patient's presenting complaint
- ☐ Changes in bowel movements
- ☐ Frequency of bowel movements
- ☐ Presence of blood/mucus in the stool
- ☐ Contacts with diarrhea
- ☐ Recent travel history
- ☐ Change in diet
- ☐ Changes in appetite (increased/decreased)
- ☐ Presence of weight loss/gain
- ☐ Presence of pain
- ☐ History of the pain
    - ☐ Site
    - ☐ Onset
    - ☐ Duration

- [ ] Intensity
- [ ] Radiation
- [ ] Character
- [ ] Exacerbating factors
- [ ] Relieving factors
- [ ] Medical history
- [ ] AIDS-associated illnesses, past/present
- [ ] Hospital admissions
- [ ] Surgical history
- [ ] Current medications
- [ ] Sexual history
  - [ ] Sexual orientation
  - [ ] Sexual activity
  - [ ] History of sexually transmitted diseases
  - [ ] Practice of safe sex
  - [ ] Partners' HIV status
  - [ ] Knowledge of AIDS transmission and the natural progression of the disease
- [ ] Family history
  - [ ] Heart disease
  - [ ] Diabetes
  - [ ] Thyroid disease
  - [ ] Cancer
  - [ ] Others
- [ ] Social history
  - [ ] Smoking
  - [ ] Alcohol
  - [ ] Other drug use (in particular, injectable drugs)

Physical Examination Checklist

- [ ] Overall assessment
- [ ] Vitals
  - [ ] Temperature—assess for fever
  - [ ] Pulse—assess for tachycardia

☐ Blood pressure
☐ Respirations
☐ Examine the abdomen
  ☐ Inspect
  ☐ Auscultate
  ☐ Light palpation
  ☐ Deep palpation
  ☐ Assess for organomegaly (palpation and percussion)
  ☐ Assess for muscular rigidity
  ☐ Assess for rebound tenderness
☐ Perform a complete physical examination if time permits to assess for other features of AIDS

Differential Diagnosis

1. Bacterial dysentery
2. Viral dysentery
3. Parasitic dysentery
4. Medication side effect
5. Colonic neoplasm

Follow-Up

1. Stool culture and examination for ova, cysts, and parasites
2. CD4+ cell count
3. Encourage practicing safe sex
4. Encourage the use of anti-retroviral medications
5. Patient education regarding the possible risk of transmission to other individuals through sexual contact, contact with bodily fluids, shared needles, and so on. Also discuss possible risks of transmission through occupation, sports, accidents, and so forth.

ALCOHOLIC NEUROPATHY

A 40-year-old patient is seen in the emergency department. He reports that he was recently hospitalized following a collapse at work. He was discharged from the hospital 3 days ago. He is now complaining of pain in his hands, his feet, and his right leg. He also complains of loss of sensation in these areas as well. The patient further reports that he has had these symptoms in the past some years ago and at that time they were relieved with bed rest and fluids. The patient describes the pain as a burning sensation. He denies fever, his appetite is good, and he has not noticed any weight loss. He has no significant medical history. He denies the use of cigarettes. He reluctantly admits that he drinks approximately one bottle of vodka a day and has done so for the past 15 years.

Patient History Checklist

- ☐ Patient's name
- ☐ Patient's age
- ☐ Patient's address
- ☐ Patient's occupation (details of all current and previous occupations with any toxin or chemical exposure)
- ☐ Patient's presenting complaint
- ☐ History of the pain
  - ☐ Site
  - ☐ Onset
  - ☐ Duration
  - ☐ Intensity
  - ☐ Radiation
  - ☐ Character
  - ☐ Exacerbating factors
  - ☐ Relieving factors
- ☐ Changes in bowel movements
- ☐ Changes in appetite (increased/decreased)
- ☐ Weight gain/loss

- ☐ Dietary history
- ☐ Medical history
- ☐ Hospital admissions
- ☐ Surgical history
- ☐ Medications
- ☐ Family history
  - ☐ Heart disease
  - ☐ Diabetes
  - ☐ Thyroid disease
  - ☐ Cancer
  - ☐ Others
- ☐ Social history
  - ☐ Smoking
  - ☐ Alcohol
  - ☐ Other drug use

Physical Examination Checklist

- ☐ Overall assessment
- ☐ Vitals
  - ☐ Temperature
  - ☐ Pulse
  - ☐ Blood pressure
  - ☐ Respirations
- ☐ Evaluate mental status
  - ☐ Orientation to person, place, and time
  - ☐ Level of consciousness
  - ☐ Short-term memory
  - ☐ Long-term memory
  - ☐ Observe the patient's gait and speech
- ☐ Examine the head
  - ☐ Assess for masses, ecchymosis, lacerations, tenderness
- ☐ Examine the ears
  - ☐ Assess the external ear canal for fluid drainage
  - ☐ Assess the tympanic membranes
- ☐ Examine all cranial nerves (I–XII)

- [ ] Examine the sensory system
  - [ ] Check for pain and crude touch in all parts of the body
  - [ ] Romberg's test
  - [ ] Proprioception at fingers and toes
  - [ ] Vibratory sense
  - [ ] Stereognosis
  - [ ] Graphesthesia
  - [ ] 2-point discrimination
  - [ ] Point localization
  - [ ] Extinction
- [ ] Examine the motor system
  - [ ] Inspect the motor system for atrophy, fasciculations, and involuntary movements
  - [ ] Palpate all limbs for muscle tone
  - [ ] Check all major muscle groups for power
  - [ ] Check all reflexes
    - [ ] Abdominal
    - [ ] Plantar
    - [ ] Biceps
    - [ ] Triceps
    - [ ] Brachioradialis
    - [ ] Knee
    - [ ] Ankle
- [ ] Examine the cerebellum
  - [ ] Ask the patient to walk in a straight line, heel to toe
  - [ ] Ask the patient to walk in a straight line on his/her heels
  - [ ] Ask the patient to walk in a straight line on his/her toes
  - [ ] Ask the patient to perform the finger–nose test
  - [ ] Ask the patient to perform the knee–heel–shin test
  - [ ] Check for dysdiadochokinesia
- [ ] If time permits, perform a full abdominal examination to assess for signs of malnutrition and liver disease/failure

Differential Diagnosis

1. Diabetic neuropathy
2. Cerebrovascular accident
3. Vascular insufficiency
4. Toxic neuropathy
5. Carpal tunnel syndrome (hand involvement only)

Follow-Up

1. Referral to counseling and/or agency such as Alcoholics Anonymous
2. Dietary counseling
3. Liver function tests (LFTs)
4. Protime/Prothrombin time (PT/PTT)
5. Ultrasound of the liver
6. Complete blood count (CBC)
7. Doppler studies
8. Electromyography (EMG)
9. Vitamin supplementation

APPENDICITIS

A 14-year-old female presents complaining of abdominal pain. She reports that the pain started 1 day ago at the umbilical area but has since localized to the right lower quadrant. She has vomited 3 times since the onset of the pain and reports that she has had a fever (maximum temperature 101.8°F). She denies any past or current sexual activity and reports that her periods are normal and she has not experienced any vaginal discharge. She has been healthy in the past and never has been admitted to the hospital. She denies any ill contacts and has not traveled recently. There is no significant family history.

Patient History Checklist

☐ Patient's name
☐ Patient's age
☐ Patient's address
☐ Patient's occupation
☐ Patient's presenting complaint
☐ Absence/presence of abdominal pain
☐ History of the pain
  ☐ Site
  ☐ Onset
  ☐ Duration
  ☐ Intensity
  ☐ Radiation
  ☐ Character
  ☐ Exacerbating factors
  ☐ Relieving factors
☐ Changes in bowel movements
☐ Changes in appetite (increased/decreased)
☐ Changes in menstrual cycle
☐ Frequency of micturition
☐ Presence of dysuria

- ☐ Presence of nocturia
- ☐ Presence of hematuria
- ☐ Medical history
- ☐ Hospital admissions
- ☐ Surgical history
- ☐ Medications
- ☐ Family history
  - ☐ Heart disease
  - ☐ Diabetes
  - ☐ Thyroid disease
  - ☐ Cancer
  - ☐ Others
- ☐ Social history
  - ☐ Smoking
  - ☐ Alcohol
  - ☐ Other drug use
- ☐ Sexual history
  - ☐ Age of menarche
  - ☐ Frequency of periods
  - ☐ Last menstrual period
  - ☐ Duration of periods
  - ☐ Presence of dysmenorrhea
  - ☐ Age of menopause (if relevant)
  - ☐ Sexual activity
  - ☐ History of sexually transmitted diseases
  - ☐ Practice of safe sex
  - ☐ Number of pregnancies/outcomes of pregnancies

Physical Examination Checklist

- ☐ Overall assessment
- ☐ Vitals
  - ☐ Temperature—assess for fever
  - ☐ Pulse—assess for tachycardia or bradycardia
  - ☐ Blood pressure—assess for hypotension
  - ☐ Respirations

☐ Examine the abdomen
  ☐ Inspect
  ☐ Auscultate
  ☐ Light palpation
  ☐ Deep palpation
  ☐ Assess for organomegaly (palpation and percussion)
  ☐ Assess for muscular rigidity
  ☐ Assess for referred rebound tenderness
  ☐ Rovsing's sign
  ☐ Assess for rebound tenderness
  ☐ Psoas sign
  ☐ Obturator sign
  ☐ Cutaneous hyperesthesia
☐ Indicate to the patient that you would like to perform a digital rectal examination but will not do so during this examination

Differential Diagnosis

1. Urinary tract infection
2. Pelvic inflammatory disease (female)
3. Ectopic pregnancy (female)
4. Ovarian cyst (female)
5. Ovarian torsion (female)
6. Cholecystitis
7. Gastroenteritis
8. Viral disease with pelvic lymphadenitis

Follow-Up

■ Digital rectal examination (DRE)
■ Beta human chorionic gonadotrophin (β-HCG) (female)
■ Pelvic examination (female)
■ Complete blood count (CBC)
■ Urinalysis (U/A)

ASTHMA

A 16-year-old male is brought to the outpatient department by his mother. His mother states that he has been asthmatic since the age of 2. The patient usually suffers 2–3 asthma attacks per year. He is allergic to cat dander and also to dust. Three days ago he began to experience shortness of breath accompanied by some wheezing. He has been using his inhaler since that time with some relief. He states that he is still short of breath on exertion and is still waking up a few times in the night feeling uncomfortable and having to use his inhaler. He has no other significant medical history and his family history is unremarkable.

Patient History Checklist

- ☐ Patient's name
- ☐ Patient's age
- ☐ Patient's address
- ☐ Patient's occupation
- ☐ Patient's presenting complaint
- ☐ Duration of symptoms
- ☐ Presence of cough (productive/nonproductive)
- ☐ Presence of fever
- ☐ Shortness of breath
- ☐ Severity of the symptoms
- ☐ Relieving factors
- ☐ Aggravating factors
- ☐ Medications used during this acute episode/effect of medications used
- ☐ Presence of chest pain
- ☐ Presence of rhinorrhea
- ☐ Allergies
- ☐ Frequency of attacks
- ☐ Prior hospitalizations for asthma
- ☐ Medical history

- ☐ Hospital admissions
- ☐ Surgical history
- ☐ Medications
- ☐ Family history
  - ☐ Asthma/allergies
  - ☐ Heart disease
  - ☐ Diabetes
  - ☐ Thyroid disease
  - ☐ Cancer
  - ☐ Others
- ☐ Social history
  - ☐ Smoking
  - ☐ Alcohol
  - ☐ Other drug use
  - ☐ Occupational exposure to dust inhalation

Physical Examination Checklist

- ☐ Overall assessment
- ☐ Vitals
  - ☐ Temperature
  - ☐ Pulse—assess for tachycardia
  - ☐ Blood pressure
  - ☐ Respirations—assess for tachypnea
- ☐ Examine the face
  - ☐ Assess mucous membranes for the presence of cyanosis or pallor
- ☐ Examine the extremities
  - ☐ Assess for clubbing
  - ☐ Assess for cyanosis
- ☐ Examine the neck
  - ☐ Assess for lymphadenopathy
  - ☐ Assess for use of accessory muscles of respiration
  - ☐ Assess the position of the trachea
- ☐ Respiratory system—examine the thorax

- ☐ Inspect
  - ☐ Size
  - ☐ Shape
  - ☐ Symmetry
  - ☐ Movement
  - ☐ Deformities of the ribs
  - ☐ Deformities of the spine
  - ☐ Scars
- ☐ Palpate
  - ☐ Tenderness
  - ☐ Excursion
  - ☐ Tactile fremitus
  - ☐ Chest dimensions
  - ☐ Position of the diaphragm
- ☐ Percuss
  - ☐ All areas comparing side to side
  - ☐ Diaphragm excursion (left)
  - ☐ Diaphragm excursion (right)
- ☐ Auscultate
  - ☐ All areas comparing side to side
  - ☐ Breath sounds
  - ☐ Vocal resonance
  - ☐ Whispering pectoriloquy
  - ☐ Aegophony

Differential Diagnosis

1. Viral upper respiratory tract infection
2. Pneumonia
3. Laryngo-tracheo-bronchitis
4. Anxiety
5. Foreign body aspiration

Follow-Up

1. Chest x-ray (CXR)
2. Spirometry
3. Pulmonary function testing (PFTs)
4. Complete blood count (CBC)
5. Sputum sample
6. Arterial blood gases (ABGs)

CARPAL TUNNEL SYNDROME

A 30-year-old female is seen in the office. She complains that she developed a pain in her right hand 6 months ago. Since the onset of the pain she has noticed that the pain has been becoming gradually worse. She describes the pain as a burning type of pain which affects all of the fingers in her right hand with the exception of her little finger. The pain travels up her arm almost to the shoulder. She states that the pain is bad during the day and worse at night, occasionally waking her up. She has also noticed that she has pain in other areas which include her shoulders, neck, and back. The pain in these areas feels different from the pain in her hand and is not as severe. She has never experienced morning stiffness. She has been healthy in the past and has never been hospitalized for any reason. She lives with her husband and their two children. She is employed as a typist in a hospital. She denies the use of alcohol and cigarettes.

Patient History Checklist

- ☐ Patient's name
- ☐ Patient's age
- ☐ Patient's address
- ☐ Patient's occupation
- ☐ Patient's presenting complaint
- ☐ Absence/presence of pain
- ☐ History of the pain
    - ☐ Site
    - ☐ Onset
    - ☐ Duration
    - ☐ Intensity
    - ☐ Radiation
    - ☐ Character
    - ☐ Exacerbating factors

- ☐ Relieving factors
- ☐ Medications used to relieve symptoms
- ☐ Presence of pain on movement
- ☐ Swelling of the affected area
- ☐ Redness of the affected area
- ☐ Presence of nausea/vomiting
- ☐ Presence of fatigue
- ☐ Presence of fever
- ☐ Previous episodes of symptoms
- ☐ History of trauma
- ☐ History of recent surgery
- ☐ History of repetitive activities—occupation, sports, recreational
- ☐ Medical history
- ☐ Hospital admissions
- ☐ Surgical history
- ☐ Family history
  - ☐ Heart disease
  - ☐ Diabetes
  - ☐ Thyroid disease
  - ☐ Cancer
  - ☐ Others
  - ☐ Medications
- ☐ Social history
  - ☐ Smoking
  - ☐ Alcohol
  - ☐ Other drug use

Physical Examination Checklist

- ☐ Overall assessment—pay particular attention to signs of endocrine disease (acromegaly, hypothyroidism, diabetes mellitus)
- ☐ Vitals
  - ☐ Temperature
  - ☐ Pulse
  - ☐ Blood pressure
  - ☐ Respirations

- ☐ Examine the extremities (bilaterally)
  - ☐ Inspect upper extremities
    - ☐ Symmetry
    - ☐ Deformities
    - ☐ Muscle wasting
    - ☐ Swellings
    - ☐ Areas of erythema
    - ☐ Active range of motion
  - ☐ Palpate upper extremities
    - ☐ Temperature
    - ☐ Tenderness
    - ☐ Masses
- ☐ Assess passive range of motion
- ☐ Assess mobility of the wrist joints
- ☐ Assess mobility of the finger joints
- ☐ Check for pain and crude touch in the hands
- ☐ Check for light touch in the hands
- ☐ Perform Phalen's test
- ☐ Check for Tinel's sign
- ☐ Examine the cervical spine
  - ☐ Symmetry
  - ☐ Deformities
  - ☐ Swelling
  - ☐ Redness
  - ☐ Active range of motion
  - ☐ Palpate
    - ☐ Temperature
    - ☐ Tenderness
    - ☐ Masses
- ☐ Check reflexes
  - ☐ Biceps
  - ☐ Triceps
  - ☐ Brachioradialis

Differential Diagnosis

1. Tendonitis
2. Trauma
3. Sprain
4. Rheumatoid arthritis
5. Cervical spine disorder

Follow-Up

1. Nonsteroidal anti-inflammatory drugs (NSAIDs)
2. Wrist splint
3. Rheumatoid factor (RF)
4. Erythrocyte sedimentation rate (ESR)
5. Blood glucose level
6. Thyroid stimulating hormone (TSH)
7. Free thyroxine (T_4)/free triiodothyroxine (T_3)
8. Skull x-ray (if endocrine cause is suspected)
9. Beta human chorionic gonadotrophin (β-HCG) (if pregnancy is suspected)
10. Surgery

CATARACTS

A 74-year-old female is seen in the clinic complaining of increasing difficulty reading. She first noticed that she was having some changes in her vision about 6 months ago and since that time the problem seems to have become worse. She complains that at the onset of the symptoms she found that her vision seemed cloudy. Her vision appeared hazy. Since that time she has found that her ability to distinguish colors has worsened. She complains that the vision in her left eye seems to be much worse than the vision in her right eye. She has been wearing reading glasses for the past 30 years and her vision has remained steady until recently. She is able to do her daily household chores without difficulty; however, finds that her night vision is affected due to the hazy appearance of objects. She also has a problem with bright lights, as they seem to cause halos around objects. Her medical history is significant for depression for which she has been treated for the past 10 years. She lives with her husband and their two cats. She denies the use of cigarettes and drinks three to four glasses of white wine a day.

Patient History Checklist

☐ Patient's name
☐ Patient's age
☐ Patient's address
☐ Patient's occupation
☐ Patient's presenting complaint
☐ Duration of symptoms
☐ Presence of headaches
☐ Presence of blurred vision
☐ Previous problems with vision
☐ Presence of cloudy vision
☐ Sensitivity to light
☐ Difficulty with night vision

☐ Presence of eye pain
☐ Dryness of the eyes
☐ Presence of dizziness
☐ Ability to perform daily activities
☐ Use of glasses
☐ Medical history
☐ Hospital admissions
☐ Surgical history
☐ Medications
☐ Family history
  ☐ Heart disease
  ☐ Diabetes
  ☐ Thyroid disease
  ☐ Cancer
  ☐ Others
☐ Social history
  ☐ Smoking
  ☐ Alcohol
  ☐ Other drug use

Physical Examination Checklist

☐ Overall assessment
☐ Vitals
  ☐ Temperature
  ☐ Pulse
  ☐ Blood pressure
  ☐ Respirations
☐ Examine the eyes
  ☐ Alignment
  ☐ Lid swelling
  ☐ Lid lesions
  ☐ Lid retraction
  ☐ Check visual acuity
  ☐ Check peripheral visual fields
  ☐ Examine anterior chamber

☐ Examine the iris
☐ Examine the pupils
☐ Opthalmoscopic examination
   ☐ Obstruction to light by lens
   ☐ Retinal hemorrhages
   ☐ Microaneurysms
   ☐ Neovascularization
   ☐ Hard exudates

Differential Diagnosis

1. Macular degeneration
2. Glaucoma
3. Presbyopia
4. Alcohol use
5. Diabetic retinopathy
6. Medications

Follow-Up

1. Referral to ophthalmologist
2. Stronger glasses or bifocals
3. Recommend appropriate lighting in home
4. Surgery

CHOLECYSTITIS

A 45-year-old male is seen in the emergency department complaining of severe abdominal pain. The pain is located in the upper abdomen, midline to slightly right-sided. He first had the pain upon waking up in the morning. He describes the pain as agonizing and "coming and going." He experiences the pain every 10 minutes. He denies fever. He has not had any constipation or diarrhea. His appetite was good until the onset of the pain this morning and since that time he has had nothing to eat. He has had a few similar episodes over the past year but the pain has never been as severe. He avoids fatty foods as they tend to make his stomach upset and the previous episodes have occurred following a greasy meal. He has no significant medical history. He has noticed that there has been a change in the color of his urine since waking up this morning, in that the urine is darker in color and appears frothy and bubbly. His family history is significant for gallbladder disease. Both his sister and his mother have had gallbladder surgery in the past. The only other significant family history is diabetes. The patient drinks approximately 4 beers a night and smokes approximately 15 cigarettes a day.

Patient History Checklist

☐ Patient's name
☐ Patient's age
☐ Patient's address
☐ Patient's occupation
☐ Patient's presenting complaint
☐ Absence/presence of abdominal pain
☐ History of the pain
    ☐ Site
    ☐ Onset
    ☐ Duration
    ☐ Intensity
    ☐ Radiation

- [ ] Character
- [ ] Exacerbating factors
- [ ] Relieving factors
- [ ] Changes in bowel movements
- [ ] Change in color of stool
- [ ] Changes in appetite (increased/decreased)
- [ ] Changes in diet
- [ ] Presence of nausea/vomiting
- [ ] Change in color of urine
- [ ] Previous episodes
- [ ] Medical history
- [ ] Hospital admissions
- [ ] Surgical history
- [ ] Medications
- [ ] Family history
  - [ ] Gallbladder disease
  - [ ] Heart disease
  - [ ] Diabetes
  - [ ] Thyroid disease
  - [ ] Cancer
  - [ ] Others
- [ ] Social history
  - [ ] Smoking
  - [ ] Alcohol
  - [ ] Other drug use

Physical Examination Checklist

- [ ] Overall assessment
- [ ] Vitals
  - [ ] Temperature—assess for fever
  - [ ] Pulse
  - [ ] Blood pressure—assess for hypotension
  - [ ] Respirations
- [ ] Examine the abdomen
  - [ ] Inspect

☐ Auscultate
☐ Light palpation
☐ Deep palpation
☐ Assess for organomegaly (palpation and percussion)
☐ Assess for muscular rigidity
☐ Assess for rebound tenderness
☐ Murphy's sign
☐ Boas' sign
☐ Indicate to the patient that you would like to perform a rectal examination but will not do so during this examination

Differential Diagnosis

1. Pancreatitis
2. Gastroesophageal reflux
3. Alcoholic gastritis
4. Hepatitis
5. Esophageal spasm
6. Appendicitis

Follow-Up

1. Digital rectal examination (DRE)
2. Ultrasound
3. Endoscopic retrograde cholangiopancreatography (ERCP)
4. Pain control
5. Surgery
6. Lipid profile

COCAINE ABUSE

A 29-year-old male is seen in the outpatient clinic. He states that he has been feeling unwell for the past 6 months. He is vague about his symptoms and obtaining a history proves to be a difficult task. On further questioning, the patient becomes very agitated and defensive. He is currently unemployed and lives alone. When questioned about drug and alcohol use the patient becomes further agitated and demands that something be done to make him feel better. When questioned still further, the patient admits that he has been using cocaine for the past year and has been drinking daily for the past 3 years. He states that he is ready for a change in his lifestyle, but requires help in doing so. He currently drinks approximately one bottle of vodka per day and smokes 2 packs of cigarettes per day. He is unsure exactly how much cocaine he uses per day but states that it is a lot.

Patient History Checklist

- ☐ Patient's name
- ☐ Patient's age
- ☐ Patient's address
- ☐ Patient's occupation
- ☐ Patient's presenting complaint
- ☐ Duration of symptoms
- ☐ Social history
  - ☐ Smoking (how much?)
  - ☐ Alcohol (how much?)
  - ☐ Drug use (specific drugs, including method of use)
  - ☐ Family situation
  - ☐ Work situation
  - ☐ Ability to function at work
  - ☐ Ability to function at home
  - ☐ Presence of support system
- ☐ Presence of fatigue

- ☐ Presence of irritability
- ☐ Difficulty concentrating
- ☐ Difficulty sleeping
- ☐ Presence of palpitations
- ☐ Loss of appetite
- ☐ Presence of weight loss/gain
- ☐ Medical history
- ☐ Hospital admissions
- ☐ Surgical history
- ☐ Medications
- ☐ Sexual history
  - ☐ Number of sexual partners
  - ☐ History of sexually transmitted diseases
  - ☐ Use of condoms
  - ☐ HIV status
- ☐ Family history
  - ☐ Drug abuse
  - ☐ Depression
  - ☐ Psychiatric illnesses
  - ☐ Heart disease
  - ☐ Diabetes
  - ☐ Thyroid disease
  - ☐ Cancer
  - ☐ Others

Physical Examination Checklist

- ☐ Overall assessment
- ☐ Vitals
  - ☐ Temperature
  - ☐ Pulse—assess for tachycardia
  - ☐ Blood pressure
  - ☐ Respirations
- ☐ Examine the neck
  - ☐ Examine JVP wave pattern
  - ☐ Measure the JVP
  - ☐ Carotid arteries—assess for bruits

- [ ] Cardiovascular system
  - [ ] Inspect the precordium
    - [ ] Shape
    - [ ] Scars
    - [ ] Pulses
    - [ ] Apex
  - [ ] Palpate the precordium
    - [ ] Tenderness
    - [ ] Pulses
    - [ ] Apex
    - [ ] Thrill
    - [ ] Heaves
  - [ ] Percuss the heart borders
  - [ ] Auscultate with the bell
    - [ ] Aortic area
    - [ ] Pulmonic area
    - [ ] Erb's point
    - [ ] Tricuspid area
    - [ ] Apex (mitral) area
  - [ ] Auscultate with the diaphragm
    - [ ] Aortic area
    - [ ] Pulmonic area
    - [ ] Erb's point
    - [ ] Tricuspid area
    - [ ] Apex (mitral) area
  - [ ] Auscultate with the bell—patient in left lateral recumbent position
  - [ ] Auscultate with the bell—patient in aortic position
- [ ] Examine the abdomen
  - [ ] Inspect
  - [ ] Auscultate
  - [ ] Light palpation
  - [ ] Deep palpation
  - [ ] Assess for organomegaly (palpation and percussion)
  - [ ] Assess for muscular rigidity
  - [ ] Assess for rebound tenderness

☐ Assess for signs of liver failure (hepatomegaly, spider angiomas, gynecomastia, caput medusa, ascites)
☐ If time permits, perform an examination of the central nervous system, paying particular attention to the pupils
☐ Perform a complete physical examination if time permits to assess for other features of drug/alcohol abuse

Differential Diagnosis

1. Alcohol abuse
2. Depression
3. HIV
4. Anxiety
5. Thyrotoxicosis
6. Anemia

Follow-Up

1. Drug rehabilitation center
2. Counseling
3. Support groups
4. Antidepressant medication
5. Evaluate HIV status
6. Thyroid stimulating hormone (TSH)
7. Free thyroxine (T_4)/ free triiodothyroxine (T_3)
8. Complete blood count (CBC)

CONCUSSION

A 17-year-old female is seen in the emergency department. She complains of feeling lightheaded and dizzy for the past 2 days. She reports that 2 days ago at school she had become very dizzy and nauseated. She does not remember exactly what happened at school, only that she woke up lying on the floor. When she "came to" there were some students around her but no one claimed to have seen her fall. She has a large bruise on the back of her head which is tender to touch. She also reports that over the past 2 days she has been feeling very irritable and fatigued. She denies any visual disturbances or numbness, and has no difficulty walking. She is continuing to experience dizziness and headaches. Her medical history is unremarkable.

Patient History Checklist

☐ Patient's name
☐ Patient's age
☐ Patient's address
☐ Patient's occupation
☐ Patient's presenting complaint
☐ Absence/presence pain
☐ History of the pain
    ☐ Site
    ☐ Onset
    ☐ Duration
    ☐ Intensity
    ☐ Radiation
    ☐ Character
    ☐ Exacerbating factors
    ☐ Relieving factors
    ☐ Medications used to relieve symptoms
☐ Presence of dizziness
☐ Presence of nausea/vomiting

- ☐ Presence of fatigue
- ☐ Sexual history
  - ☐ Age of menarche
  - ☐ Frequency of periods
  - ☐ Last menstrual period
  - ☐ Duration of periods
  - ☐ Presence of dysmenorrhea
  - ☐ Frequency of sexual intercourse
  - ☐ History of sexually transmitted diseases
  - ☐ Presence of vaginal discharge
  - ☐ Presence of dyspareunia
  - ☐ Number of pregnancies/outcomes of pregnancies
  - ☐ Number of abortions
  - ☐ Reasons for abortions
- ☐ Presence of irritability
- ☐ Difficulty concentrating
- ☐ Difficulty sleeping
- ☐ Previous episode of symptoms
- ☐ Incontinence of urine
- ☐ Incontinence of feces
- ☐ Bite injury to tongue
- ☐ History of trauma
- ☐ Medical history
- ☐ Hospital admissions
- ☐ Surgical history
- ☐ Medications

Physical Examination Checklist

- ☐ Overall assessment
- ☐ Vitals
  - ☐ Temperature—assess for fever
  - ☐ Pulse
    - ☐ Assess for tachycardia or bradycardia
    - ☐ Assess for arrhythmias
  - ☐ Blood pressure—assess for hypotension

- [ ] Respirations
- [ ] Evaluate mental status
  - [ ] Orientation to person, place, and time
  - [ ] Level of consciousness
  - [ ] Short-term memory
  - [ ] Long-term memory
  - [ ] Observe the patient's gait and speech
- [ ] Examine the head
  - [ ] Assess for masses, ecchymosis, lacerations, tenderness
  - [ ] Examine the tongue for bite injury
- [ ] Examine the ears
  - [ ] Assess the external ear canal for fluid drainage
  - [ ] Assess the tympanic membranes
- [ ] Examine all cranial nerves (I–XII)
- [ ] Examine the sensory system
  - [ ] Check for pain and crude touch in all parts of the body
  - [ ] Romberg's test
  - [ ] Proprioception at fingers and toes
  - [ ] Vibratory sense
  - [ ] Stereognosis
  - [ ] Graphesthesia
  - [ ] 2-point discrimination
  - [ ] Point localization
  - [ ] Extinction
- [ ] Examine the motor system
  - [ ] Inspect the motor system for atrophy, fasciculations, and involuntary movements
  - [ ] Palpate all limbs for muscle tone
  - [ ] Check all major muscle groups for power
  - [ ] Check all reflexes
    - [ ] Abdominal
    - [ ] Plantar
    - [ ] Biceps
    - [ ] Triceps
    - [ ] Brachioradialis
    - [ ] Knee
    - [ ] Ankle

☐ Examine the cerebellum
  ☐ Ask the patient to walk in a straight line, heel to toe
  ☐ Ask the patient to walk in a straight line on his/her heels
  ☐ Ask the patient to walk in a straight line on his/her toes
  ☐ Ask the patient to perform the finger–nose test
  ☐ Ask the patient to perform the knee–heel–shin test
  ☐ Check for dysdiadochokinesia

Differential Diagnosis

1. Grand mal seizure
2. Postural hypotension
3. Diabetes mellitus
4. Substance abuse
5. Anemia
6. Pregnancy
7. Intracranial mass

Follow-Up

1. Observation
2. Head x-ray
3. Computed tomography scan (CT)
4. Electroencephalogram (EEG)
5. Fasting blood glucose level
7. Electrocardiogram (ECG)
8. Beta human chorionic gonadotrophin (β-HCG) (female)
9. Toxicology (drug screening)

CONGESTIVE HEART FAILURE

A 65-year-old female is seen in the emergency department. She is complaining of feeling short of breath for the past 3 weeks. She has noticed that the shortness of breath is becoming worse. She reports that she has never experienced similar symptoms in the past. She also complains of a persistent cough over the same period of time. She describes her sputum as pink and frothy. She has difficulty sleeping at night due to the shortness of breath and finds that it helps her if she sits up in the bed or sits in her recliner to sleep. Her medical history is significant for hypertension; however, she reports that she has not been to see her primary care physician for quite a few years and is not currently taking any medication for the blood pressure. She denies the use of cigarettes or alcohol.

Patient History Checklist

☐ Patient's name
☐ Patient's age
☐ Patient's address
☐ Patient's occupation
☐ Patient's presenting complaint
☐ Duration of symptoms
☐ Presence of cough (productive/nonproductive)
☐ Presence of fever
☐ Shortness of breath
☐ Severity of the symptoms
☐ Previous episodes of symptoms
☐ Swelling of the extremities
☐ Changes in diet/salt intake
☐ Presence of palpitations
☐ Relieving factors
☐ Aggravating factors

- [ ] Medications used during this acute episode/effect of medications used
- [ ] Presence of chest pain
- [ ] Allergies
- [ ] Risk factors
  - [ ] Family history
  - [ ] Hypertension
  - [ ] Diabetes
  - [ ] Previous heart condition
  - [ ] Smoking
  - [ ] Alcohol
  - [ ] Exercise
  - [ ] Occupation
  - [ ] Stress at present
- [ ] Medical history
- [ ] Hospital admissions
- [ ] Surgical history
- [ ] Medications

Physical Examination Checklist

- [ ] Overall assessment
- [ ] Vitals
  - [ ] Temperature—assess for fever
  - [ ] Pulse—assess for arrhythmias
  - [ ] Blood pressure—assess for hypertension
  - [ ] Respirations
- [ ] Examine the face
  - [ ] Assess mucous membranes for the presence of cyanosis or pallor
- [ ] Examine the extremities
  - [ ] Assess for clubbing
  - [ ] Assess for cyanosis
  - [ ] Assess for pitting edema
- [ ] Examine the neck
  - [ ] Examine JVP wave pattern
  - [ ] Measure the JVP

- ☐ Carotid arteries—assess for bruits
- ☐ Assess for use of accessory muscles of respiration
- ☐ Assess the position of the trachea
- ☐ Respiratory system—examine the thorax
  - ☐ Inspect
    - ☐ Size
    - ☐ Shape
    - ☐ Symmetry
    - ☐ Movement
    - ☐ Deformities of the ribs
    - ☐ Deformities of the spine
    - ☐ Scars
  - ☐ Palpate
    - ☐ Tenderness
    - ☐ Excursion
    - ☐ Tactile fremitus
    - ☐ Chest dimensions
    - ☐ Position of the diaphragm
  - ☐ Percuss
    - ☐ All areas comparing side to side
    - ☐ Diaphragm excursion (left)
    - ☐ Diaphragm excursion (right)
  - ☐ Auscultate
    - ☐ All areas comparing side to side
    - ☐ Breath sounds
    - ☐ Adventitious sounds
    - ☐ Vocal resonance
    - ☐ Whispering pectoriloquy
    - ☐ Aegophony
- ☐ Cardiovascular system
  - ☐ Inspect the precordium
    - ☐ Shape
    - ☐ Scars
    - ☐ Pulses
    - ☐ Apex

- ☐ Palpate the precordium
  - ☐ Tenderness
  - ☐ Pulses
  - ☐ Apex
  - ☐ Thrills
  - ☐ Heaves
- ☐ Percuss the heart borders
- ☐ Auscultate with the bell
  - ☐ Aortic area
  - ☐ Pulmonic area
  - ☐ Erb's point
  - ☐ Tricuspid area
  - ☐ Apex (mitral) area
- ☐ Auscultate with the diaphragm
  - ☐ Aortic area
  - ☐ Pulmonic area
  - ☐ Erb's point
  - ☐ Tricuspid area
  - ☐ Apex (mitral) area
- ☐ Auscultate with the bell—patient in left lateral recumbent position
- ☐ Auscultate with the bell—patient in aortic position

Differential Diagnosis

1. Cardiac arrhythmia
2. Pneumonia
3. Asthma
4. Anemia

Follow-Up

1. Chest x-ray (CXR)
2. Electrocardiogram (ECG)
3. Cardiac enzymes (CK, CK-MB, Troponin)
4. Diuretics
5. Echocardiogram (EcHO)
6. Stress test
7. Lipid profile
8. Pulmonary function tests (PFTs)
9. Arterial blood gases (ABGs)

DEMENTIA

A 68-year-old female is brought to the family physician by her husband. He has noticed that she is having increasing difficulty with her memory. Mainly her short-term memory seems to be affected. She is able to recall events that happened many years ago in detail, but is often unable to recall something that happened earlier the same day or earlier in the week. She denies this and states that her memory is just fine. Her husband also has been noticing that she often calls objects by the wrong names. She has been healthy in the past. Her medical history is significant for hypothyroidism which she was diagnosed with 10 years ago. The only medication she uses is thyroxine for the hypothyroidism. She has no allergies. She denies the use of alcohol or any other drug use.

Patient History Checklist

- ☐ Patient's name
- ☐ Patient's age
- ☐ Patient's address
- ☐ Patient's occupation
- ☐ Patient's presenting complaint
- ☐ Duration of symptoms
- ☐ Presence of memory loss
- ☐ Presence of forgetfulness
- ☐ Difficulty concentrating
- ☐ Presence of fatigue
- ☐ Presence of irritability
- ☐ Difficulty sleeping
- ☐ Loss of appetite
- ☐ Presence of weight loss/gain
- ☐ Presence of hallucinations
- ☐ Altered level of consciousness
- ☐ Presence of delusions

- ☐ Previous episode of symptoms
- ☐ Heat intolerance
- ☐ Palpitations
- ☐ Anxiety
- ☐ Cold intolerance
- ☐ Medical history
- ☐ Hospital admissions
- ☐ Surgical history
- ☐ Medications
- ☐ Family history
  - ☐ Psychiatric illnesses
  - ☐ Heart disease
  - ☐ Diabetes
  - ☐ Thyroid disease
  - ☐ Cancer
  - ☐ Others
- ☐ Social history
  - ☐ Smoking
  - ☐ Alcohol
  - ☐ Other drug use
  - ☐ Family situation
  - ☐ Work situation
  - ☐ Ability to function at work
  - ☐ Ability to function at home
  - ☐ Presence of support system
  - ☐ Ability to perform daily tasks
  - ☐ Ability to reside safely at home

Physical Examination Checklist

- ☐ Overall assessment
- ☐ Vitals
  - ☐ Temperature
  - ☐ Pulse
    - ☐ Assess for tachycardia or bradycardia
    - ☐ Assess for arrhythmias

☐ Blood pressure
☐ Respirations
☐ Evaluate mental status
  ☐ Orientation to person, place, and time
  ☐ Level of consciousness
  ☐ Short-term memory
  ☐ Long-term memory
  ☐ Observe the patient's gait and speech
☐ Examine the head
  ☐ Assess for masses, ecchymosis, lacerations, tenderness
☐ Examine the ears
  ☐ Assess the external ear canal for fluid drainage
  ☐ Assess the tympanic membranes
☐ Examine all cranial nerves (I–XII)
☐ Examine the sensory system
  ☐ Check for pain and crude touch in all parts of the body
  ☐ Romberg's test
  ☐ Proprioception at fingers and toes
  ☐ Vibratory sense
  ☐ Stereognosis
  ☐ Graphesthesia
  ☐ 2-point discrimination
  ☐ Point localization
  ☐ Extinction
☐ Examine the motor system
  ☐ Inspect the motor system for atrophy, fasciculations, and involuntary movements
  ☐ Palpate all limbs for muscle tone
  ☐ Check all major muscle groups for power
☐ Check all reflexes
  ☐ Abdominal
  ☐ Plantar
  ☐ Biceps
  ☐ Triceps
  ☐ Brachioradialis
  ☐ Knee
  ☐ Ankle

☐ Examine the cerebellum
  ☐ Ask the patient to walk in a straight line, heel to toe
  ☐ Ask the patient to walk in a straight line on his/her heels
  ☐ Ask the patient to walk in a straight line on his/her toes
  ☐ Ask the patient to perform the finger–nose test
  ☐ Ask the patient to perform the knee–heel–shin test
  ☐ Check for dysdiadochokinesia

Differential Diagnosis

1. Alzheimer's dementia
2. Multi-infarct dementia
3. Delirium
4. Hypothyroidism
5. Depression
6. Thyroxine overuse

Follow-Up

1. Thyroid stimulating hormone (TSH)
2. Free thyroxine (T_4)/free triiodothyroxine (T_3)
3. Complete blood count (CBC)
4. Urinalysis (U/A)
5. Electrolytes
6. Venereal Disease Research Laboratory test (VDRL)
7. Chest x-ray (CXR)
8. Electrocardiogram (ECG)
9. Evaluation of home situation and safety in the home

DEPRESSION

A 27-year-old male is seen by his primary care physician. He states that he has "not been feeling quite right" for the past 3 weeks. He has no interest in his usual activities. He is usually an avid baseball player but has not been motivated to play lately. He is employed as a bank teller and usually really enjoys his job, but over the last three weeks has called in sick to work 7 times because he states that he just wasn't in the mood to work. He reports that he has been losing some weight, his appetite is poor, and he is not sleeping well. He finds that he is able to fall asleep at night with no problem. However, he wakes up around 3:00 in the morning and is unable to fall back asleep. He recently broke up with his long-term girlfriend but when questioned about this he states, "She's probably better off; I'm not good enough for her anyway." He has one brother with a history of depression. The rest of his family history is unremarkable. His medical history is also unremarkable.

Patient History Checklist

☐ Patient's name
☐ Patient's age
☐ Patient's address
☐ Patient's occupation
☐ Patient's presenting complaint
☐ Duration of symptoms
☐ Presence of fatigue
☐ Presence of irritability
☐ Difficulty concentrating
☐ Difficulty sleeping
☐ Presence of early morning waking
☐ Loss of appetite
☐ Presence of weight loss/gain
☐ Loss of interest in sexual intercourse

☐ Loss of interest in hobbies
☐ Tearfulness
☐ Feelings of worthlessness
☐ Presence of hallucinations
☐ Presence of delusions
☐ Suicidal ideation
    ☐ Suicide plan
    ☐ Previous suicide attempts
☐ Previous episode of symptoms
☐ Medical history
☐ Hospital admissions
☐ Surgical history
☐ Medications
☐ Family history
    ☐ Depression
    ☐ Psychiatric illnesses
    ☐ Heart disease
    ☐ Diabetes
    ☐ Thyroid disease
    ☐ Cancer
    ☐ Others
☐ Social history
    ☐ Smoking
    ☐ Alcohol
    ☐ Other drug use
    ☐ Family situation
    ☐ Work situation
    ☐ Ability to function at work
    ☐ Ability to function at home
    ☐ Presence of support system

Physical Examination Checklist

☐ If time permits, perform an assessment for hypothyroidism. Also perform a full central nervous system examination

Differential Diagnosis

1. Hypothyroidism
2. Bipolar disorder
3. Alcohol abuse
4. Diabetes mellitus

Follow-Up

1. Counseling
2. Support groups
3. Antidepressant medication
4. Complete blood count (CBC)
5. Fasting blood glucose level
6. Thyroid stimulating hormone (TSH)
7. Free thyroxine (T_4)/free triiodothyroxine (T_3)

DIABETES

A 56-year-old male is seen by his primary care physician. He is a known diabetic and follows up with his physician every 3 months for care of his diabetes. He was first diagnosed with diabetes 6 years ago. He has had no diabetic complications to date and his blood sugar is well controlled. He checks his blood glucose at home 3 times per day. He has no other medical conditions and has been well in the past. He is obese, but he has been maintaining a steady weight for the past 3 years. His family history is significant for heart disease, hypertension, and diabetes. He denies the use of alcohol and cigarettes.

Patient History Checklist

- [ ] Patient's name
- [ ] Patient's age
- [ ] Patient's address
- [ ] Patient's occupation
- [ ] Patient's presenting complaint
- [ ] Presence of polyuria
- [ ] Presence of polydipsia
- [ ] Presence of excessive thirst
- [ ] Blood glucose readings at home
- [ ] Diet
- [ ] Presence of weight loss/gain
- [ ] Presence of chest pain
- [ ] Presence of shortness of breath
- [ ] Presence of peripheral edema
- [ ] Changes in vision
- [ ] Presence of lower extremity ulcers or sores
- [ ] Family history
  - [ ] Diabetes
  - [ ] Hypertension

☐ Previous heart condition
☐ Smoking
☐ Alcohol
☐ Exercise
☐ Occupation
☐ Stress at present
☐ Medical history
☐ Hospital admissions
☐ Surgical history
☐ Medications

Physical Examination Checklist

☐ Overall assessment
☐ Vitals
    ☐ Temperature
    ☐ Pulse
    ☐ Blood pressure
    ☐ Respirations
☐ Examine the eyes (especially fundoscopy)
    ☐ Cataracts
    ☐ Retinal hemorrhages
    ☐ Microaneurysms
    ☐ Neovascularization
    ☐ Hard exudates
☐ Examine the neck
    ☐ Examine JVP wave pattern
    ☐ Measure the JVP
    ☐ Carotid arteries—assess for bruits
☐ Cardiovascular system
    ☐ Inspect the precordium
        ☐ Shape
        ☐ Scars
        ☐ Pulses
        ☐ Apex
    ☐ Palpate the precordium
        ☐ Tenderness

- ☐ Pulses
- ☐ Apex
- ☐ Thrill
- ☐ Heaves
- ☐ Percuss the heart borders
- ☐ Auscultate with the bell
  - ☐ Aortic area
  - ☐ Pulmonic area
  - ☐ Erb's point
  - ☐ Tricuspid area
  - ☐ Apex (mitral) area
- ☐ Auscultate with the diaphragm
  - ☐ Aortic area
  - ☐ Pulmonic area
  - ☐ Erb's point
  - ☐ Tricuspid area
  - ☐ Apex (mitral) area
- ☐ Auscultate with the bell—patient in left lateral recumbent position
- ☐ Auscultate with the bell—patient in aortic position
- ☐ Inspect the upper and lower extremities for size and symmetry
- ☐ Examine the nails, hair, and skin
- ☐ Observe any ulcers or gangrene, taking care to examine the soles of the feet
- ☐ Palpate temperature in both the upper and the lower extremities comparing both limbs
- ☐ Palpate pulses
  - ☐ Dorsalis pedis
  - ☐ Posterior tibial
  - ☐ Popliteal
  - ☐ Femoral
  - ☐ Radial
  - ☐ Ulnar
  - ☐ Brachial
- ☐ Perform Allen's test
- ☐ Perform Buerger's test
- ☐ Check for bruits over the abdominal aorta and both the iliofemoral arteries

☐ Examine the motor system
  ☐ Inspect the motor system for atrophy, fasciculations, and involuntary movements
  ☐ Palpate all limbs for muscle tone
  ☐ Check all major muscle groups for power
  ☐ Check all reflexes
    ☐ Abdominal
    ☐ Plantar
    ☐ Biceps
    ☐ Triceps
    ☐ Brachioradialis
    ☐ Knee
    ☐ Ankle
☐ Examine the sensory system
  ☐ Check for pain and crude touch in all parts of the body
  ☐ Romberg's test
  ☐ Proprioception at fingers and toes
  ☐ Vibratory sense
  ☐ Stereognosis
  ☐ Graphesthesia
  ☐ 2-point discrimination
  ☐ Point localization
  ☐ Extinction

Differential Diagnosis

1. Diabetes insipidus
2. Urinary tract infection

Follow-Up

1. Blood glucose level
2. Glycosylated hemoglobin level (HgA1C)
3. Urinalysis (U/A)
4. Nutritional counseling
5. Diabetes education

DOMESTIC VIOLENCE

A 27-year-old female is seen in the clinic. She complains of left-sided chest pain which is particularly painful when she takes a deep breath or presses on the area. She states that she had a fall at home but is vague about the details of how the fall came about. She lives at home with her husband and their three children. She is a stay-at-home mom. When questioned about her medical history she is again vague and states that she has been healthy with the exception of some bruises, broken bones, and lacerations from previous falls. She has been admitted to the hospital 7 times in the past year for injuries. In the past she has sustained a broken jaw, a broken left fibula, and multiple rib fractures. When questioned about her married life, the patient becomes tearful and upset. She states that the only reason that she is attending the clinic is to obtain something for the pain in her side and that there are no further issues that she would like to discuss.

Patient History Checklist

☐ Patient's name
☐ Patient's age
☐ Patient's address
☐ Patient's occupation
☐ Patient's presenting complaint
☐ Presence of chest pain
☐ Site of chest pain
☐ Presence of ecchymosis
☐ Duration of symptoms
☐ Previous episode of symptoms
☐ Shortness of breath
☐ Severity of the symptoms
☐ Relieving factors

- [ ] Aggravating factors
- [ ] Medications used during this acute episode/effect of medications used
- [ ] Abuse history
  - [ ] How injury occurred
  - [ ] Presence of abuse in the home
  - [ ] History of abuse in the home
  - [ ] Frequency of abuse
  - [ ] Presence of emotional abuse
  - [ ] Presence of physical abuse
  - [ ] Presence of sexual abuse
  - [ ] Presence of child abuse in the home
  - [ ] Presence of guns in the home
  - [ ] Use of alcohol in the home
  - [ ] Use of illegal drugs in the home
  - [ ] Presence of an escape plan
- [ ] Medical history
- [ ] Hospital admissions
- [ ] Surgical history
- [ ] Medications
- [ ] Family history
  - [ ] Depression
  - [ ] Psychiatric illnesses
  - [ ] Heart disease
  - [ ] Diabetes
  - [ ] Thyroid disease
  - [ ] Cancer
  - [ ] Others
- [ ] Social history
  - [ ] Smoking
  - [ ] Alcohol
  - [ ] Other drug use
  - [ ] Family situation
  - [ ] Work situation
  - [ ] Ability to function at work
  - [ ] Ability to function at home
  - [ ] Presence of support system

Physical Examination Checklist

- ☐ Overall assessment
- ☐ Vitals
  - ☐ Temperature
  - ☐ Pulse
  - ☐ Blood pressure
  - ☐ Respirations
- ☐ Respiratory system—examine the thorax
  - ☐ Inspect
    - ☐ Size
    - ☐ Shape
    - ☐ Symmetry
    - ☐ Movement
    - ☐ Deformities of the ribs
    - ☐ Deformities of the spine
    - ☐ Scars
  - ☐ Palpate
    - ☐ Tenderness
    - ☐ Excursion
    - ☐ Tactile fremitus
    - ☐ Chest dimensions
    - ☐ Position of the diaphragm
  - ☐ Percuss
    - ☐ All areas comparing side to side
    - ☐ Diaphragm excursion (left)
    - ☐ Diaphragm excursion (right)
  - ☐ Auscultate
    - ☐ All areas comparing side to side
    - ☐ Breath sounds
    - ☐ Vocal resonance
    - ☐ Whispering pectoriloquy
    - ☐ Aegophony
- ☐ Examine the skin
  - ☐ Assess for areas of ecchymosis, lacerations, and scars
- ☐ Perform a complete physical examination if time permits to assess for other signs of physical abuse

Differential Diagnosis

1. Syncope
2. Alcohol abuse
3. Drug abuse
4. Grand mal seizures
5. Psychosis

Follow-Up

1. Pain control
2. Social worker assessment of children's safety in the home
3. Counseling
4. Support groups
5. Help hotlines
6. Domestic violence shelters
7. Psychiatric referral (if necessary)

DYSPHAGIA

A 32-year-old female is seen in the outpatient department complaining of difficulty swallowing. She reports that she has been having some difficulty swallowing for the past 3 months. The problem seems to be worsening. She complains that it is difficult to swallow both liquids and solids. She finds that sometimes after taking a bite of food she has a choking/coughing episode and feels that it is difficult to breathe. She has never experienced similar symptoms. She has no other complaints. She states that her appetite has been poor; however, she has not noticed any weight loss. She denies nausea or vomiting and has been afebrile since the onset of the symptoms. She complains that she often experiences chest pain following eating. She describes the pain as centrally located in her chest and as a burning sensation. She does not take any medications. She drinks approximately 2 glasses of wine per day and smokes approximately 15 cigarettes per day.

Patient History Checklist

- ☐ Patient's name
- ☐ Patient's age
- ☐ Patient's address
- ☐ Patient's occupation
- ☐ Patient's presenting complaint
- ☐ Presence of difficulty swallowing
- ☐ Presence of difficulty swallowing solid foods
- ☐ Presence of difficulty swallowing liquids
- ☐ Duration of symptoms
- ☐ Presence of chest pain
- ☐ History of the pain
  - ☐ Site
  - ☐ Onset
  - ☐ Duration

- ☐ Intensity
- ☐ Radiation
- ☐ Character
- ☐ Exacerbating factors
- ☐ Relieving factors
- ☐ Medications used to try to relieve the pain
- ☐ Changes in weight (loss/gain)
- ☐ Changes in bowel movements
- ☐ Changes in appetite (increased/decreased)
- ☐ Presence of melena
- ☐ Presence of hematemesis
- ☐ Presence of nausea/vomiting
- ☐ Presence of cough
- ☐ Presence of shortness of breath
- ☐ Presence of fever
- ☐ Presence of swelling in the neck
- ☐ History of psychiatric illness
- ☐ Medical history
- ☐ Hospital admissions
- ☐ Surgical history
- ☐ Medications
- ☐ Family history
  - ☐ Thyroid disease
  - ☐ Gastric ulcers
  - ☐ Heart disease
  - ☐ Diabetes
  - ☐ Cancer
  - ☐ Psychiatric illnesses
  - ☐ Others
- ☐ Social history
  - ☐ Smoking
  - ☐ Alcohol
  - ☐ Other drug use

Physical Examination Checklist

- ☐ Overall assessment
- ☐ Vitals
  - ☐ Temperature
  - ☐ Pulse
  - ☐ Blood pressure
  - ☐ Respirations
- ☐ Examine the neck
  - ☐ Assess for any swellings
  - ☐ Assess for normal thyroid gland
- ☐ Examine the abdomen
  - ☐ Inspect
  - ☐ Auscultate
  - ☐ Light palpation
  - ☐ Deep palpation
  - ☐ Assess for organomegaly (palpation and percussion)
  - ☐ Assess for muscular rigidity
  - ☐ Assess for rebound tenderness
- ☐ Cardiovascular system
  - ☐ Inspect the precordium
    - ☐ Shape
    - ☐ Scars
    - ☐ Pulses
    - ☐ Apex
  - ☐ Palpate the precordium
    - ☐ Tenderness
    - ☐ Pulses
    - ☐ Apex
    - ☐ Thrill
    - ☐ Heaves
  - ☐ Percuss the heart borders
  - ☐ Auscultate with the bell
    - ☐ Aortic area
    - ☐ Pulmonic area
    - ☐ Erb's point

- ☐ Tricuspid area
- ☐ Apex (mitral) area
- ☐ Auscultate with the diaphragm
  - ☐ Aortic area
  - ☐ Pulmonic area
  - ☐ Erb's point
  - ☐ Tricuspid area
  - ☐ Apex (mitral) area
- ☐ Auscultate with the bell—patient in left lateral recumbent position
- ☐ Auscultate with the bell—patient in aortic position
- ☐ Respiratory system—examine the thorax
  - ☐ Inspect
    - ☐ Size
    - ☐ Shape
    - ☐ Symmetry
    - ☐ Movement
    - ☐ Deformities of the ribs
    - ☐ Deformities of the spine
    - ☐ Scars
  - ☐ Palpate
    - ☐ Tenderness
    - ☐ Excursion
    - ☐ Tactile fremitus
    - ☐ Chest dimensions
    - ☐ Position of the diaphragm
  - ☐ Percuss
    - ☐ All areas comparing side to side
    - ☐ Diaphragm excursion (left)
    - ☐ Diaphragm excursion (right)
  - ☐ Auscultate
    - ☐ All areas comparing side to side
    - ☐ Breath sounds
    - ☐ Vocal resonance
    - ☐ Whispering pectoriloquy
    - ☐ Aegophony
- ☐ Indicate to the patient that you would like to perform a digital rectal examination but will not do so during this examination

Differential Diagnosis

1. Achalasia
2. Goiter
3. Abnormal relaxation of the upper esophageal sphincter
4. Esophageal webs
5. Scleroderma
6. Globus hystericus
7. Esophageal carcinoma

Follow-Up

1. Digital rectal examination (DRE)
2. Stool guiac
3. Thyroid stimulating hormone (TSH)
4. Free thyroxine (T_4)/free triiodothyroxine (T_3)
5. Complete blood count (CBC)
6. Barium swallow
7. Esophagogastroduodenoscopy (EGD)
8. Patient education regarding diet and lifestyle

ECTOPIC PREGNANCY

A 22-year-old female is seen in the outpatient clinic complaining of abdominal pain. The pain started 24 hours ago and is becoming progressively worse. She has not noticed any aggravating or relieving factors. The pain is located in the left lower quadrant and does not radiate. She rates the pain as an 8 on a scale of 1–10 with 10 being the worst pain. She denies vaginal discharge. She has not had any episodes of diarrhea or constipation and has not experienced any nausea or vomiting. Her appetite has been poor since the onset of the pain and she has been unable to sleep. She lives with her boyfriend and is employed in a restaurant as a waitress. Her last menstrual period was 5 weeks ago, but the patient states that her periods are often irregular. She is sexually active and uses condoms as a method of birth control. She never has been pregnant in the past and denies ever having any sexually transmitted diseases.

Patient History Checklist

- ☐ Patient's name
- ☐ Patient's age
- ☐ Patient's address
- ☐ Patient's occupation
- ☐ Patient's presenting complaint
- ☐ Absence/presence of abdominal pain
- ☐ History of the pain
  - ☐ Site
  - ☐ Onset
  - ☐ Duration
  - ☐ Intensity
  - ☐ Radiation
  - ☐ Character

- ☐ Exacerbating factors
- ☐ Relieving factors
- ☐ Changes in bowel movements
- ☐ Changes in appetite (increased/decreased)
- ☐ Presence of nausea/vomiting
- ☐ Changes in menstrual cycle
- ☐ Frequency of micturition
- ☐ Presence of dysuria
- ☐ Presence of nocturia
- ☐ Presence of hematuria
- ☐ Sexual history
  - ☐ Age of menarche
  - ☐ Frequency of periods
  - ☐ Last menstrual period
  - ☐ Duration of periods
  - ☐ Presence of dysmenorrhea
  - ☐ Frequency of sexual intercourse
  - ☐ Number of sexual partners
  - ☐ History of sexually transmitted diseases
  - ☐ Presence of vaginal discharge
  - ☐ Presence of dyspareunia
  - ☐ Number of pregnancies/outcomes of pregnancies
  - ☐ Number of abortions
  - ☐ Reasons for abortions
- ☐ Presence of weight loss/gain
- ☐ Changes in breasts
- ☐ Changes in skin pigmentation
- ☐ Partner's details
  - ☐ Age
  - ☐ Occupation
  - ☐ History of sexually transmitted diseases
  - ☐ Number of sexual partners
  - ☐ Number of children, if any
- ☐ Medical history
- ☐ Hospital admissions
- ☐ Surgical history
- ☐ Medications

- ☐ Family history
    - ☐ Heart disease
    - ☐ Diabetes
    - ☐ Hypertension
    - ☐ Cancer
    - ☐ Others
- ☐ Social history
    - ☐ Smoking
    - ☐ Alcohol
    - ☐ Other drug use
    - ☐ Family situation

Physical Examination Checklist

- ☐ Overall assessment
- ☐ Vitals
    - ☐ Temperature—assess for fever
    - ☐ Pulse—assess for tachycardia or bradycardia
    - ☐ Blood pressure—assess for hypotension
    - ☐ Respirations
- ☐ Examine the abdomen
    - ☐ Inspect
    - ☐ Auscultate
    - ☐ Light palpation
    - ☐ Deep palpation
    - ☐ Assess for organomegaly (palpation and percussion)
    - ☐ Assess for muscular rigidity
    - ☐ Assess for referred rebound tenderness
    - ☐ Rovsing's sign
    - ☐ Assess for rebound tenderness
    - ☐ Psoas sign
    - ☐ Obturator sign
    - ☐ Cutaneous hyperesthesia
- ☐ Indicate to the patient that you would like to perform a pelvic examination including vaginal cultures but will not do so during this examination

Differential Diagnosis

1. Pelvic inflammatory disease (female)
2. Appendicitis
3. Ovarian cyst (female)
4. Ovarian torsion (female)
5. Urinary tract infection

Follow-Up

1. Bimanual pelvic examination
2. Beta human chorionic gonadotrophin (β-HCG) (female)
3. Vaginal cultures (female)
4. Abdominal ultrasound
5. Complete blood count (CBC)
6. Urinalysis (U/A)

FEVER IN AN INFANT

A 21-year-old woman is seen in the outpatient clinic. She is 5 weeks postpartum and is doing well. She states that the reason for her visit is not for herself but rather for her infant whom she has not brought with her at this time. She is worried about germs in the clinic so decided to leave the infant at home for fear that he would come into contact with infection. The infant she reports is not doing too well. He has been healthy since birth until yesterday when he developed a fever. She reports that he has been feeding well and gaining weight until the onset of the fever. He is both breast and bottle fed. His bowel movements have been regular. The maximum temperature (rectally) at home was 102.5°F. He has had one episode of vomiting and has not been eating well since the onset. She has noticed that he has had fewer wet diapers than usual over the past 24 hours. The infant lives at home with his mother, his father, and 1 sibling (3 years old), and they are all well. She has not noticed any skin rashes. His delivery was a normal vaginal delivery and there were no complications during the pregnancy.

Patient History Checklist

☐ Patient's name
☐ Patient's age
☐ Patient's address
☐ Patient's presenting complaint
☐ Maximum temperature
☐ Presence of weight loss/gain
☐ Changes in bowel movements
☐ Changes in appetite (increased/decreased)
☐ Number of wet diapers
☐ Presence of skin rash
☐ Irritability/lethargy
☐ Presence of cough

- [ ] Presence of shortness of breath
- [ ] Ill contacts (especially household members)
- [ ] Birth history
  - [ ] Duration of pregnancy
  - [ ] Complications during the pregnancy
  - [ ] Weeks of gestation at delivery
  - [ ] Frequency of prenatal care
  - [ ] Duration of labor
  - [ ] Complications during delivery
  - [ ] Immunizations up to date
  - [ ] Mother's prior pregnancies
  - [ ] Outcomes of any prior pregnancies
- [ ] Family history of diseases (mother, father, and siblings)
  - [ ] Heart disease
  - [ ] Diabetes
  - [ ] Thyroid disease
  - [ ] Sickle cell disease
  - [ ] Psychiatric disorders
  - [ ] Sexually transmitted diseases
- [ ] Diet (breast or bottle fed)
- [ ] Social history
  - [ ] Living situation
  - [ ] Pets in the home
  - [ ] Smoking in the home

Physical Examination Checklist

- [ ] Advise mother to return to the clinic with the infant for a full assessment. If the history suggests that the infant requires hospitalization, advise the mother to take the infant to the emergency department immediately for evaluation.

Differential Diagnosis

1. Bacterial infection, including:
   Bacteremia
   Pneumonia
   Urinary tract infection
   Pyelonephritis
   Otitis media
   Meningitis
2. Viral infection
3. Dehydration
4. Diarrhea

Follow-Up

1. Full physical examination
2. Complete blood count (CBC)
3. Blood cultures
4. Urinalysis (U/A)
5. Urine culture
6. Assessment of hydration/rehydration needs
7. Lumbar puncture (LP) (if necessary)
8. Antibiotics (if necessary)

GASTRIC ULCER

A 42-year-old male is seen in the clinic. He complains of having a burning pain in his abdomen. He reports that he has been having the pain for the past 3 months. The pain comes on gradually about 1 hour following a meal. The pain is associated with nausea most of the time and on quite a few occasions he has vomited while experiencing the pain. He states that although it is unpleasant to vomit, his pain is greatly relieved by vomiting. He reports that he has noticed a significant weight loss over the past 3 months and attributes this to the fact that he now avoids a lot of his favorite foods as they seem to make the pain worse. His favorite foods are hot wings and spicy curries. His medical history is unremarkable. He denies the use of cigarettes but does admit that he drinks a 6-pack of beer a day after work. His family history is significant for alcohol abuse by both his father and one of his brothers.

Patient History Checklist

☐ Patient's name
☐ Patient's age
☐ Patient's address
☐ Patient's occupation
☐ Patient's presenting complaint
☐ Absence/presence of abdominal pain
☐ History of the pain
   ☐ Site
   ☐ Onset
   ☐ Duration
   ☐ Intensity
   ☐ Radiation
   ☐ Character
   ☐ Exacerbating factors
   ☐ Relieving factors
   ☐ Medications used to try to relieve the pain

☐ Presence of weight loss/gain
☐ Changes in bowel movements
☐ Changes in appetite (increased/decreased)
☐ Presence of melena
☐ Presence of hematemesis
☐ Medical history
☐ Hospital admissions
☐ Surgical history
☐ Medications
☐ Family history
    ☐ Gastric ulcers
    ☐ Heart disease
    ☐ Diabetes
    ☐ Thyroid disease
    ☐ Cancer
    ☐ Others
☐ Social history
    ☐ Smoking
    ☐ Alcohol
    ☐ Other drug use

Physical Examination Checklist

☐ Overall assessment
☐ Vitals
    ☐ Temperature
    ☐ Pulse—assess for tachycardia
    ☐ Blood pressure—assess for hypotension
    ☐ Respirations
☐ Examine the abdomen
    ☐ Inspect
    ☐ Auscultate
    ☐ Light palpation
    ☐ Deep palpation
    ☐ Assess for organomegaly (palpation and percussion)

☐ Assess for muscular rigidity
☐ Assess for rebound tenderness
☐ Perform a full cardiovascular examination if time permits
☐ Indicate to the patient that you would like to perform a digital rectal examination but will not do so during this examination

Differential Diagnosis

1. Hiatus hernia
2. Gastroesophageal reflux
3. Alcoholic gastritis
4. Gastric neoplasm
5. Esophageal spasm
6. Angina

Follow-Up

1. Digital rectal examination
2. Stool guiac
3. Complete blood count (CBC)
4. Esophagogastroduodenoscopy (EGD)
5. Electrocardiogram (ECG)

GOUT

A 43-year-old male is seen in the clinic. He is very concerned about a pain that he has recently experienced in his foot. He states that the pain started approximately 10 days ago while he was visiting family in New York. The pain came on very suddenly overnight, localized to his right big toe. The toe was also warm to the touch and appeared very red. He states that at the time he also felt slightly feverish and nauseated. He was seen in the emergency department in New York at the time of onset and an x-ray was done which did not reveal any abnormalities. The pain and swelling was severe for approximately 1 week and then resolved. He noticed that the skin over his big toe peeled off. He has had no further symptoms since that time. He had a similar episode 2 years ago and has come to the clinic to see if he can find out what is going on and if the source of these episodes of pain can be determined.

Patient History Checklist

☐ Patient's name
☐ Patient's age
☐ Patient's address
☐ Patient's occupation
☐ Patient's presenting complaint
☐ Absence/presence of pain
☐ History of the pain
    ☐ Site
    ☐ Onset
    ☐ Duration
    ☐ Intensity
    ☐ Radiation
    ☐ Character
    ☐ Exacerbating factors

☐ Relieving factors
☐ Medications used to relieve symptoms
☐ Presence of pain on movement
☐ Swelling of the affected area
☐ Redness of the affected area
☐ Presence of nausea/vomiting
☐ Presence of fatigue
☐ Presence of fever
☐ Presence of morning stiffness
☐ Previous episodes of symptoms
☐ History of trauma
☐ History of recent surgery
☐ Use of diuretics
☐ History of alcoholic binge drinking
☐ History of unusual exercise
☐ History of exposure to toxic heavy metals, particularly lead
☐ Medical history
☐ Hospital admissions
☐ Surgical history
☐ Medications
☐ Family history
   ☐ Heart disease
   ☐ Diabetes
   ☐ Thyroid disease
   ☐ Cancer
   ☐ Others
☐ Social history
   ☐ Smoking
   ☐ Alcohol
   ☐ Other drug use

Physical Examination Checklist

☐ Overall assessment
☐ Vitals
    ☐ Temperature
    ☐ Pulse
    ☐ Blood pressure
    ☐ Respirations
☐ Observe patient's gait
☐ Examine the extremities
    ☐ Inspect lower extremities
        ☐ Symmetry
        ☐ Deformities
        ☐ Swellings
        ☐ Areas of erythema
    ☐ Palpate lower extremities
        ☐ Temperature
        ☐ Tenderness
        ☐ Masses
☐ Assess mobility of hip joints
☐ Assess mobility of knee joints
☐ Assess mobility of ankle joints
☐ Assess mobility of finger joints
☐ Assess mobility of foot joints
☐ Perform a full cardiovascular examination if time permits

Differential Diagnosis

1. Trauma
2. Osteomyelitis
3. Osteoarthritis
4. Stress fracture
5. Cellulitis

Follow-Up

1. Serum uric acid level
2. Joint aspiration and synovial fluid microscopy
3. X-ray (of affected joint)
4. Complete blood count (CBC)
5. Blood urea nitrogen level (BUN) and blood creatinine level
6. Lipid profile
7. Nonsteroidal anti-inflammatory drugs (NSAIDs)
8. Colchicine

HEARING LOSS

A 32-year-old female is seen by her primary care physician. She complains that she has noticed that she is having difficulty hearing. She first noticed that there was a problem 2 weeks ago when she realized that she was having difficulty hearing the television when no one else seemed to be having difficulty. She denies ever having any similar problems in the past. She has not done anything unusual over the past few weeks such as swimming or diving. She does not use cotton swabs in her ears. She has not noticed any drainage from the ears. She has been afebrile and denies any pain associated with her ears. Her medical history is significant for asthma which is well controlled with albuterol.

Patient History Checklist

☐ Patient's name
☐ Patient's age
☐ Patient's address
☐ Patient's occupation
☐ Patient's presenting complaint
☐ Duration of symptoms
☐ Presence of ear pain
☐ Presence of drainage from ears
☐ Presence of fever
☐ History of previous episodes
☐ Presence of ringing in the ears
☐ Use of cotton swabs
☐ Presence of dizziness
☐ Presence of headaches
☐ Presence of nausea
☐ Presence of vomiting
☐ Medical history
☐ Hospital admissions
☐ Surgical history

- ☐ Medications
- ☐ Family history
  - ☐ Heart disease
  - ☐ Diabetes
  - ☐ Thyroid disease
  - ☐ Cancer
  - ☐ Others
- ☐ Social history
  - ☐ Smoking
  - ☐ Alcohol
  - ☐ Other drug use

Physical Examination Checklist

- ☐ Overall assessment
- ☐ Vitals
  - ☐ Temperature
  - ☐ Pulse
  - ☐ Blood pressure
  - ☐ Respirations
- ☐ Inspect the external ears
  - ☐ Deformities
  - ☐ Discharge
  - ☐ Symmetry
  - ☐ Lesions
  - ☐ Inflammation
- ☐ Palpate
  - ☐ Tragus
  - ☐ Auricle
  - ☐ Mastoid process
- ☐ Inspect the external canal with an ear speculum
- ☐ Inspect the tympanic membrane
  - ☐ Color
  - ☐ Cone of light
  - ☐ Handle of malleus
  - ☐ Incus

☐ Perforations
☐ Retractions
☐ Perform the whisper test
☐ Perform Weber's test
☐ Perform Rinne's test

Differential Diagnosis

1. Cerumen impaction
2. Otitis media
3. Labyrinthitis
4. Sinus infection
5. Meniere's disease

Follow-Up

1. Follow-up and treatment will be based on the findings of the physical examination

HIP FRACTURE

A 77-year-old female is transferred to the hospital from her assisted living home. The staff at the home found the patient lying on the floor of her bathroom. The patient was confused upon being found and could not give any information as to how or at what time the fall had taken place. While transferring the patient to the hospital, a large ecchymosis was noted on her left buttock and her left posterior thigh. She complained of feeling some pain around her left buttock and was unable to bear weight at all on the left side. Her medical history is significant for hypertension, diabetes, osteoporosis, and mild congestive heart failure. She takes a variety of medications for these conditions. She has smoked cigarettes for the past 60 years, approximately 1 pack per day. She denies the use of alcohol. Her meals are provided by the home where she resides and the staff report that her appetite is fairly good and she eats a wide variety of foods.

Patient History Checklist

- ☐ Patient's name
- ☐ Patient's age
- ☐ Patient's address
- ☐ Patient's occupation
- ☐ Patient's presenting complaint
- ☐ Absence/presence of pain
- ☐ History of the pain
  - ☐ Site
  - ☐ Onset
  - ☐ Duration
  - ☐ Intensity
  - ☐ Radiation
  - ☐ Character
  - ☐ Exacerbating factors
  - ☐ Relieving factors
  - ☐ Medications used to relieve symptoms

- [ ] History of fall/injury
- [ ] Time of fall/injury
- [ ] Loss of consciousness at time of fall
- [ ] Presence of dizziness at time of fall
- [ ] Previous falls
- [ ] Previous fractures
- [ ] Difficulty with vision
- [ ] Presence of pain on movement
- [ ] Swelling of the affected area
- [ ] Redness of the affected area
- [ ] Presence of ecchymosis
- [ ] Presence of nausea/vomiting
- [ ] Presence of fatigue
- [ ] Medical history
- [ ] Hospital admissions
- [ ] Surgical history
- [ ] Medications (including vitamin supplements)
- [ ] Age of menopause
- [ ] Number of children
- [ ] Family history
  - [ ] Heart disease
  - [ ] Diabetes
  - [ ] Thyroid disease
  - [ ] Cancer
  - [ ] Others
- [ ] Social history
  - [ ] Smoking
  - [ ] Alcohol
  - [ ] Other drug use

Physical Examination Checklist

- [ ] Overall assessment
- [ ] Vitals
  - [ ] Temperature
  - [ ] Pulse—assess for bradycardia

☐ Blood pressure—assess for postural hypotension
☐ Respirations
☐ Examine the extremities (bilaterally)
   ☐ Inspect upper extremities
      ☐ Symmetry
      ☐ Deformities
      ☐ Swellings
      ☐ Areas of erythema and/or ecchymoses
   ☐ Palpate upper extremities
      ☐ Temperature
      ☐ Tenderness
      ☐ Masses
   ☐ Inspect lower extremities
      ☐ Symmetry
      ☐ Deformities
      ☐ Swellings
      ☐ Areas of erythema
   ☐ Palpate lower extremities
      ☐ Temperature
      ☐ Tenderness
      ☐ Masses
☐ Assess mobility of hip joints
☐ Assess mobility of knee joints
☐ Assess mobility of ankle joints
☐ Assess mobility of finger joints
☐ Assess mobility of foot joints
☐ Assess for external rotation of hip joint
☐ Check all reflexes
   ☐ Abdominal
   ☐ Plantar
   ☐ Biceps
   ☐ Triceps
   ☐ Brachioradialis
   ☐ Quadriceps
   ☐ Knee
   ☐ Ankle

☐ Palpate temperature in both the upper and the lower extremities comparing both limbs
☐ Palpate pulses
  ☐ Dorsalis pedis
  ☐ Posterior tibial
  ☐ Popliteal
  ☐ Femoral
  ☐ Radial
  ☐ Ulnar
  ☐ Brachial
☐ If time permits, perform a full cardiovascular examination

Differential Diagnosis

Hip Pain:

1. Trauma
2. Bursitis
3. Osteoarthritis

Fall:

1. Cardiac arrythmia
2. Postural hypotension
3. Anemia

Follow-Up

1. Hip x-ray
2. Pain control (care regarding mental confusion and sedation is required)
3. Electrocardiogram (ECG)
4. Complete blood count (CBC)
5. Orthopedic consultation

HYPERTENSION

A 45-year-old male is seen in the clinic for follow-up of his hypertension. He was initially found to be hypertensive 5 years ago. He currently takes only one medication for control of his blood pressure. His blood pressure has been well controlled since the time of diagnosis and the patient is very compliant with both medication and regular checkups. He has no other significant medical history. He is mildly obese, but has maintained a steady weight since the time of his diagnosis. He eats a healthy diet and is aware of his salt intake. He was previously a smoker, but quit smoking at the time of his diagnosis and has remained a nonsmoker since that time. He lives at home with his wife and their 3 children. His family history is significant for thyroid disease and heart disease.

Patient History Checklist

☐ Patient's name
☐ Patient's age
☐ Patient's address
☐ Patient's occupation
☐ Patient's presenting complaint
☐ Compliance with medications
☐ Patient's blood pressures
☐ Presence of weight loss/gain
☐ Revision of patient's diet
☐ Presence of headaches
☐ Presence of dizziness
☐ Presence of changes in vision
☐ Presence of chest pain
☐ Risk factors
　☐ Family history
　☐ Hypertension
　☐ Diabetes

☐ Previous heart condition
☐ Smoking
☐ Alcohol
☐ Exercise
☐ Occupation
☐ Stress at present
☐ Medical history
☐ Hospital admissions
☐ Surgical history
☐ Medications

Physical Examination Checklist

☐ Overall assessment
☐ Vitals
  ☐ Temperature
  ☐ Pulse
  ☐ Blood pressure—assess for hypertension
  ☐ Respirations
☐ Examine the neck
  ☐ Examine JVP wave pattern
  ☐ Measure the JVP
  ☐ Carotid arteries—assess for bruits
☐ Cardiovascular system
  ☐ Inspect the precordium
    ☐ Shape
    ☐ Scars
    ☐ Pulses
    ☐ Apex
  ☐ Palpate the precordium
    ☐ Tenderness
    ☐ Pulses
    ☐ Apex
    ☐ Thrill
    ☐ Heaves

- [ ] Percuss the heart borders
- [ ] Auscultate with the bell
  - [ ] Aortic area
  - [ ] Pulmonic area
  - [ ] Erb's point
  - [ ] Tricuspid area
  - [ ] Apex (mitral) area
- [ ] Auscultate with the diaphragm
  - [ ] Aortic area
  - [ ] Pulmonic area
  - [ ] Erb's point
  - [ ] Tricuspid area
  - [ ] Apex (mitral) area
- [ ] Auscultate with the bell—patient in left lateral recumbent position
- [ ] Auscultate with the bell—patient in aortic position
- [ ] Examine the eyes
  - [ ] Alignment
  - [ ] Lid swelling
  - [ ] Lid lesions
  - [ ] Lid retraction
  - [ ] Check visual acuity
  - [ ] Check peripheral visual fields
  - [ ] Examine anterior chamber
  - [ ] Examine the iris
  - [ ] Examine the pupils
- [ ] Ophthalmoscopic examination
  - [ ] Retinal hemorrhages
  - [ ] Microaneurysms
  - [ ] Neovascularization
  - [ ] Hard exudates
- [ ] A full abdominal examination should be performed if time permits

Differential Diagnosis

1. Renal disease
2. Pheochromocytoma
3. Primary aldosteronism
4. Cocaine abuse

Follow-Up

1. Review and continue antihypertensive medication(s)
2. Urinalysis (U/A)
3. Lipid profile
4. Referral to ophthalmologist for checkup
5. Encourage healthy lifestyles (eg, cigarette cessation if applicable, dietary counseling, weight loss, decreased salt intake, increased vegetables in diet, exercise)

HYPERTHYROIDISM

A 23-year-old female presents with complaints of weight loss, diarrhea, and a change in her menstrual cycle. She first noticed these symptoms approximately 4 to 5 months ago. She also has been experiencing some feelings of anxiety accompanied by palpitations. She states that she has been feeling very warm despite the cold weather outside. She has no significant medical history. Her appetite has been good and she reports that she is sleeping well. She does not smoke cigarettes and denies the use of alcohol. Her family history is only significant for thyroid disease.

Patient History Checklist

☐ Patient's name
☐ Patient's age
☐ Patient's address
☐ Patient's occupation
☐ Patient's presenting complaint
☐ Character of the stool
☐ Frequency of bowel movements
☐ Absence/presence of blood/mucus in the stool
☐ Absence/presence of abdominal pain
☐ Changes in appetite (increased/decreased)
☐ History of weight loss
☐ Fatigue
☐ Sweating
☐ Heat intolerance
☐ Palpitations
☐ Anxiety
☐ Changes in menstrual cycle
☐ Changes in the eyes
☐ Swellings in the neck
☐ History of rash on the lower extremities
☐ History of vomiting

☐ Medical history
☐ Hospital admissions
☐ Surgical history
☐ Medications
☐ Family history
  ☐ Thyroid disease
  ☐ Heart disease
  ☐ Diabetes
  ☐ Cancer
  ☐ Others
☐ Social history
  ☐ Smoking
  ☐ Alcohol
  ☐ Other drug use

Physical Examination Checklist

☐ Overall assessment
☐ Vitals
  ☐ Temperature—assess for fever
  ☐ Pulse
    ☐ Assess for tachycardia
    ☐ Assess for rapid bounding pulses
  ☐ Blood pressure—assess for increased systolic and decreased diastolic pressures (widened pulse pressure)
  ☐ Respirations
☐ Examine the eyes
  ☐ Check pupillary size
  ☐ Assess for lid retraction
  ☐ Assess for lid lag
  ☐ Assess for exopthalmos
  ☐ Assess for extraocular muscle weakness
☐ Examine the neck
  ☐ Assess for any swellings
  ☐ Assess for normal thyroid gland
☐ Cardiovascular system

- [ ] Assess for atrial fibrillation
- [ ] Assess for tachycardia
- [ ] Assess for an accentuated S1
- [ ] Assess for systolic ejection murmur
- [ ] Examine the extremities
  - [ ] Assess for excess diaphoresis of the hands
  - [ ] Assess for proximal muscle weakness
  - [ ] Assess for tremor
  - [ ] Assess for brisk tendon reflexes
  - [ ] Assess for pretibial myxedema (swelling and discoloration of the skin on the anterior lower extremities)

Differential Diagnosis

1. Anxiety disorder
2. Bipolar disorder
3. Anorexia nervosa/bulimia
4. Intestinal parasitosis
5. Drug (cocaine) abuse

Follow-Up

1. Thyroid stimulating hormone (TSH)
2. Free thyroxine (T_4)/free triiodothyroxine (T_3)
3. Ultrasound of the thyroid gland
4. Stool culture and stool for ova, cysts, and parasites
5. Radionuclide uptake scan of the thyroid gland

HYPOTHYROIDISM

A 48-year-old female presents to the outpatient clinic complaining of fatigue. She reports that the fatigue began several months ago. She states that she has also been feeling "a bit depressed" recently and finds that she is having some difficulty concentrating. On further questioning, she tells you that she also has been constipated over the past few months and has gained approximately 16 lbs despite noticing a decrease in her appetite. She has noticed that her hair has become brittle and finds that her skin is very dry. She has no significant medical history. She lives at home with her husband and their 2 children and is a stay-at-home mom.

Patient History Checklist

- ☐ Patient's name
- ☐ Patient's age
- ☐ Patient's address
- ☐ Patient's occupation
- ☐ Patient's presenting complaint
- ☐ Duration of symptoms
- ☐ Weight gain (how much and over what period of time)
- ☐ Fatigue
- ☐ Psychiatric evaluation
  - ☐ Loss of interest/difficulty concentrating
  - ☐ Agitation
  - ☐ Feelings of worthlessness
  - ☐ Delusions/hallucinations
  - ☐ Suicidal ideation
- ☐ Frequency of bowel movements
- ☐ Constipation
- ☐ Swelling around eyes
- ☐ Swelling of the lower extremities
- ☐ Changes in appetite (increased/decreased)

- ☐ Changes in sleep patterns
- ☐ Cold intolerance
- ☐ Difficulty swallowing
- ☐ Changes in menstrual cycle
- ☐ Hair changes
- ☐ Voice changes
- ☐ History of treatment for hyperthyroidism
- ☐ Swellings in neck
- ☐ Medical history, including any psychiatric illness
- ☐ Hospital admissions
- ☐ Surgical history
- ☐ Medications
- ☐ Family history
  - ☐ Thyroid disease
  - ☐ Heart disease
  - ☐ Diabetes
  - ☐ Cancer
  - ☐ Psychiatric disorders
  - ☐ Others
- ☐ Social history
  - ☐ Smoking
  - ☐ Alcohol
  - ☐ Other drug use (especially lithium)

Physical Examination Checklist

- ☐ Overall assessment
- ☐ Vitals
  - ☐ Temperature—assess for hypothermia
  - ☐ Pulse—assess for bradycardia
  - ☐ Blood pressure—assess for decreased systolic and increased diastolic pressures
  - ☐ Respirations
- ☐ Examine the face
  - ☐ Assess for facial swelling
  - ☐ Assess for coarse, dry skin

☐ Assess for swelling of the tongue
☐ Assess for thinning of the scalp hair and eyebrows (laterally)
☐ Examine the eyes
   ☐ Assess for periorbital puffiness
   ☐ Assess for thickening of the eyelids
☐ Examine the neck
   ☐ Assess for any swellings
   ☐ Assess for normal thyroid gland
☐ Examine the cardiovascular system
   ☐ Assess for diminished heart sounds
   ☐ Assess for bradycardia
☐ Examine the extremities
   ☐ Assess for swelling of the hands
   ☐ Assess for muscle weakness
   ☐ Assess for hypoactive tendon reflexes with a slow relaxation phase

Differential Diagnosis

1. Depression
2. Bipolar disorder
3. Lithium therapy
4. Anemia

Follow-Up

1. Thyroid stimulating hormone (TSH)
2. Free thyroxine (T_4)/free triiodothyroxine (T_3)
3. Ultrasound of the thyroid gland
4. Complete blood count (CBC)

IMPOTENCE

A 52-year-old male is seen in the clinic. He complains that he has been feeling very tired lately and is concerned about the control of his diabetes. He has been diabetic for the past 5 years. He checks his blood glucose twice a day and the usual range is from 100–250 mmol/dL. On further questioning he admits that he has been feeling depressed lately because he has been unable to have intercourse with his wife. It has been several months since he has been able to sustain an erection and he has not managed to have penetrative intercourse with his wife for the past 5–6 months. He states that he still desires intercourse with his wife and feels that his increasing anxiety regarding this problem is probably contributing to making the problem worse. He has also noticed that upon waking up in the morning he no longer has morning erections.

Patient History Checklist

- ☐ Patient's name
- ☐ Patient's age
- ☐ Patient's address
- ☐ Patient's occupation
- ☐ Patient's presenting complaint
- ☐ Presence of fatigue
- ☐ Presence of irritability
- ☐ Difficulty concentrating
- ☐ Difficulty sleeping
- ☐ Presence of early morning waking
- ☐ Loss of appetite
- ☐ Presence of weight loss/gain
- ☐ Loss of interest in sexual intercourse with wife or with other partners, if applicable
- ☐ Absence of morning erections
- ☐ Loss of interest in hobbies
- ☐ Tearfulness

☐ Suicidal ideation
☐ Previous episode of symptoms
☐ Medical history
☐ Hospital admissions
☐ Surgical history
☐ Medications (especially antihypertensives and diabetic drugs)
☐ Family history
   ☐ Depression
   ☐ Psychiatric illnesses
   ☐ Heart disease
   ☐ Diabetes
   ☐ Thyroid disease
   ☐ Cancer
   ☐ Others
☐ Social history
   ☐ Smoking
   ☐ Alcohol
   ☐ Other drug use
   ☐ Family situation
   ☐ Wife's reaction to impotence

Physical Examination Checklist

☐ If a physical examination is required, perform an assessment of the patient's diabetes
☐ Indicate to the patient that you would like to examine his genitalia but will not do so during this examination

Differential Diagnosis

1. Anxiety/depression
2. Drug use
3. Multiple sclerosis
4. Tertiary syphilis

Follow-Up

1. Genital examination
2. Venereal Disease Research Laboratory test (VDRL)
3. Diabetes counseling
4. Diabetes management
5. Blood glucose level
6. Glycosylated hemoglobin level (HgA1C)
7. Medication to achieve erection

INFERTILITY

A 34-year-old female presents concerning her inability to conceive. She reports that she and her husband have been trying to conceive a child for the past few years. She previously took the birth control pill but stopped using it 6 years ago. Since that time she and her husband have not used any form of contraceptive. Her inability to conceive was first investigated a few years ago when she complained of some leaking from her breasts. She has only had 2 periods since stopping the pill 6 years ago. Her last period was 4 months ago. She has been treated in the past with the fertility drug Clomid without results and is currently taking Parlodel but still has had no success. She has no significant medical history. She states that she enjoys intercourse and she and her husband have intercourse 3–4 times a week. She is requesting some help as her husband desperately wants to have a child and she has begun to feel very depressed about the whole situation.

Patient History Checklist

- Patient's name
- Patient's age
- Patient's address
- Patient's occupation
- Patient's presenting complaint
- Sexual history
    - Age of menarche
    - Frequency of periods
    - Last menstrual period
    - Duration of periods
    - Presence of dysmenorrhea
    - Frequency of sexual intercourse
    - Interest in sexual intercourse
    - History of sexually transmitted diseases
    - Presence of vaginal discharge

- ☐ Presence of dyspareunia
- ☐ Number of pregnancies/outcomes of pregnancies
- ☐ Number of abortions
- ☐ Reasons for abortions
- ☐ Presence of excess facial hair
- ☐ Presence of weight loss/gain
- ☐ Presence of nipple discharge
- ☐ Partner's details
  - ☐ Age
  - ☐ Occupation
  - ☐ History of sexually transmitted diseases
  - ☐ Number of children, if any
  - ☐ Ability to achieve vaginal penetration
  - ☐ Frequency of ejaculation
- ☐ Medical history
- ☐ Hospital admissions
- ☐ Surgical history
- ☐ Medications
- ☐ Family history
  - ☐ Siblings with children
  - ☐ Depression
  - ☐ Psychiatric illnesses
  - ☐ Heart disease
  - ☐ Diabetes
  - ☐ Thyroid disease
  - ☐ Cancer
  - ☐ Others
- ☐ Social history
  - ☐ Smoking
  - ☐ Alcohol
  - ☐ Other drug use
  - ☐ Family situation
  - ☐ Feelings of anxiety
  - ☐ Exercise

Physical Examination Checklist

☐ Overall assessment
☐ Vitals
   ☐ Temperature
   ☐ Pulse
   ☐ Blood pressure
   ☐ Respirations
☐ Observe for evidence of endocrine disorder
☐ Assess hair distribution
☐ Examine the abdomen
   ☐ Inspect
   ☐ Auscultate
   ☐ Light palpation
   ☐ Deep palpation
   ☐ Assess for organomegaly (palpation and percussion)
   ☐ Assess for pelvic abdominal masses
☐ Indicate to the patient that you would like to perform a breast examination and a pelvic examination but will not do so during this examination

Differential Diagnosis

1. Polycystic ovary disease
2. Anorexia
3. Hyperthyroidism
4. Hyperprolactinemia
5. Turner's syndrome
6. Chromosomal abnormality

Follow-Up

1. Breast examination
2. Bimanual pelvic examination
3. Complete blood count (CBC)
4. Prolactin level
5. Assessment of tubal patency
6. Follow-up of patient's partner
7. Counseling
8. Chromosome analysis

LUNG CANCER

A 49-year-old male is brought to the clinic by his wife. He has had a cough for the past 8 weeks but has been reluctant to be seen by his doctor for fear that it is "something really serious." His cough is productive with whitish sputum and is occasionally streaked with bright red blood. Three days ago he developed a pain in the left side of his chest. He states that the pain is very severe when he coughs but otherwise does not bother him much. He has been feeling generally unwell for the past year and feels that his energy level has decreased significantly. His appetite is poor and he reports that he has not been sleeping well. He wakes up in the middle of the night with aches and pains in his arms and his legs. He has been well in the past and has had no significant medical illnesses. He smokes a pack of cigarettes a day which he has been doing since he was 14 years old. He drinks occasionally at present and admits to being a heavy drinker in his teens and his 20s.

Patient History Checklist

☐ Patient's name
☐ Patient's age
☐ Patient's address
☐ Patient's occupation
☐ Patient's presenting complaint
☐ Duration of symptoms
☐ Presence of cough (productive/nonproductive)
☐ Presence of blood in the sputum
☐ Shortness of breath
☐ Presence of fever
☐ Presence of rhinorrhea
☐ Presence of chest pain
☐ History of the pain
    ☐ Site
    ☐ Onset

☐ Duration
☐ Intensity
☐ Radiation
☐ Character
☐ Exacerbating factors
☐ Relieving factors
☐ History of weight loss
☐ Presence of night sweats
☐ Medical history
☐ Hospital admissions
☐ Surgical history
☐ Medications
☐ Family history
    ☐ Cancer
    ☐ Heart disease
    ☐ Diabetes
    ☐ Thyroid disease
    ☐ Asthma/allergies
    ☐ Others
☐ Social history
    ☐ Smoking
    ☐ Alcohol
    ☐ Other drug use

Physical Examination Checklist

☐ Overall assessment
☐ Vitals
    ☐ Temperature
    ☐ Pulse—assess for tachycardia
    ☐ Blood pressure
    ☐ Respirations—assess for tachypnea
☐ Examine the face
    ☐ Assess mucous membranes for the presence of cyanosis
☐ Examine the neck
    ☐ Assess for lymphadenopathy

- ☐ Assess for use of accessory muscles
- ☐ Assess the position of the trachea
- ☐ Examine the extremities
  - ☐ Assess for clubbing
  - ☐ Assess for cyanosis
- ☐ Respiratory system—examine the thorax
  - ☐ Inspect
    - ☐ Size
    - ☐ Shape
    - ☐ Symmetry
    - ☐ Movement
    - ☐ Deformities of the ribs
    - ☐ Deformities of the spine
    - ☐ Scars
  - ☐ Palpate
    - ☐ Tenderness
    - ☐ Excursion
    - ☐ Tactile fremitus
    - ☐ Chest dimensions
    - ☐ Position of the diaphragm
  - ☐ Percuss
    - ☐ All areas comparing side to side
    - ☐ Diaphragm excursion (left)
    - ☐ Diaphragm excursion (right)
  - ☐ Auscultate
    - ☐ All areas comparing side to side
    - ☐ Breath sounds
    - ☐ Vocal resonance
    - ☐ Whispering pectoriloquy
    - ☐ Aegophony

Differential Diagnosis

1. Tuberculosis
2. Pneumonia
3. Lung abscess
4. Bronchitis

Follow-Up

1. Chest x-ray (CXR)
2. Sputum culture
3. Computed tomography scan (CT)
4. Bronchoscopy

MELENA

A 54-year-old female complains of fatigue and dizziness for the past 2 weeks. She has also been feeling very sweaty and a little faint upon standing up. She has been having loose stools for the past 2 weeks, approximately 3–5 stools per day. She has noticed that the color of her stool seems to have changed and her stool is now very dark in color, almost black. She denies ever seeing any bright red blood in her stool. She has been healthy in the past with the exception of frequent indigestion which is usually relieved by antacids or a large glass of milk. She lives with her husband and her 2 daughters, all of whom are healthy. She smokes approximately 1 pack of cigarettes per day and admits to drinking between 3–5 vodkas per day. Her family history is unremarkable.

Patient History Checklist

☐ Patient's name
☐ Patient's age
☐ Patient's address
☐ Patient's occupation
☐ Patient's presenting complaint
☐ Absence/presence of abdominal pain
☐ Pain in relation to meals
☐ Changes in bowel movements
☐ Changes in appetite (increased/decreased)
☐ Presence of weight loss/gain
☐ Presence of dizziness
☐ Presence of lightheadedness
☐ Presence of fatigue
☐ Presence of melena
☐ Presence of hematemesis
☐ History of gastric ulcers
☐ History of hemorrhoids

□ Last menstrual period
□ Medications taken to relieve symptoms
□ Medical history
□ Hospital admissions
□ Surgical history
□ Medications
□ Family history
　　□ Colon cancer
　　□ Diabetes
　　□ Thyroid disease
　　□ Others
□ Social history
　　□ Smoking
　　□ Alcohol
　　□ Other drug use

Physical Examination Checklist

□ Overall assessment
□ Vitals
　　□ Temperature
　　□ Pulse
　　□ Blood pressure
　　□ Respirations
□ Examine the abdomen
　　□ Inspect
　　□ Auscultate
　　□ Light palpation
　　□ Deep palpation
　　□ Assess for organomegaly (palpation and percussion)
　　□ Assess for muscular rigidity
　　□ Assess for rebound tenderness
□ Indicate to the patient that you would like to perform a digital rectal examination but will not do so during this examination

Differential Diagnosis

1. Colon cancer
2. Gastric ulcer
3. Hemorrhoids
4. Vaginal bleeding
5. Colonic polyps

Follow-Up

1. Digital rectal examination (DRE)
2. Stool for occult blood
3. Complete blood count (CBC)
4. Colonoscopy
5. Esophagogastroduodenoscopy (EGD)
6. Blood group and cross match

MENINGITIS

A 17-year-old female is brought to the emergency department by her parents. She has been feeling unwell for the past 2 days with some nausea, vomiting, and fatigue. Early this morning she woke up with a severe headache and a fever. She has been febrile all day with a maximum temperature of 102°F. She has continued to feel nauseated throughout the day and has had no appetite. She also reports that she has been having some pain and difficulty moving her neck since the onset of the headache. She has had no ill contacts that she is aware of. Her parents have noticed that throughout the day she has been becoming increasingly irritable. She has been healthy in the past with no prior admissions to the hospital. She denies the presence of any other symptoms.

Patient History Checklist

- ☐ Patient's name
- ☐ Patient's age
- ☐ Patient's address
- ☐ Patient's occupation
- ☐ Patient's presenting complaint
- ☐ Presence of fever (maximum temperature)
- ☐ Absence/presence pain
- ☐ History of the pain
  - ☐ Site
  - ☐ Onset
  - ☐ Duration
  - ☐ Intensity
  - ☐ Radiation
  - ☐ Character
  - ☐ Exacerbating factors
  - ☐ Relieving factors
  - ☐ Medications used to relieve symptoms
- ☐ Presence of dizziness

☐ Presence of nausea/vomiting
☐ Presence of fatigue
☐ Presence of irritability
☐ Presence of photophobia
☐ Difficulty concentrating
☐ Difficulty sleeping
☐ Previous episode of symptoms
☐ Presence of any skin rash
☐ Ill contacts
☐ Medications taken for the symptoms
☐ History of trauma
☐ Medical history
☐ Hospital admissions
☐ Surgical history
☐ Medications
☐ Family history
    ☐ Heart disease
    ☐ Diabetes
    ☐ Thyroid disease
    ☐ Cancer
    ☐ Others
☐ Social history
    ☐ Smoking
    ☐ Alcohol
    ☐ Other drug use

Physical Examination Checklist

☐ Overall assessment
☐ Vitals
    ☐ Temperature—assess for fever
    ☐ Pulse—assess for tachycardia or bradycardia
    ☐ Blood pressure
    ☐ Respirations
☐ Evaluate mental status
    ☐ Orientation to person, place, and time

- [ ] Level of consciousness
- [ ] Short-term memory
- [ ] Long-term memory
- [ ] Observe the patient's gait and speech
- [ ] Examine the skin
  - [ ] Rashes
  - [ ] Ecchymoses
- [ ] Examine the head
  - [ ] Assess for masses, ecchymosis, lacerations, tenderness
- [ ] Examine the eyes
  - [ ] Assess for papilledema
- [ ] Examine the ears
  - [ ] Assess the external ear canal for fluid drainage
  - [ ] Assess the tympanic membranes
- [ ] Assess for cervical rigidity
- [ ] Brudzinski's sign
- [ ] Kernig's sign
- [ ] Examine all cranial nerves (I–XII)

Differential Diagnosis

1. Viral meningitis
2. Bacterial meningitis
3. Encephalitis
4. Migraine
5. Tension headache

Follow-Up

1. Lumbar puncture (LP)
2. Complete blood count (CBC)
3. Blood culture
4. Computed tomography scan (CT)
5. Intravenous antibiotics

MIGRAINE

A 26-year-old female is seen by her primary care physician. She complains of a headache which started early in the morning. She describes the pain as throbbing and localized to her right side. She also reports that she is having difficulty dealing with bright lights and finds that if she lies still in a dark room the pain subsides slightly. She has vomited twice since the onset of the pain. She has had many of these headaches in the past. The first time that she ever experienced a headache similar to this one was at the age of 14. She has about 3–4 such headaches per year and finds that they are closely related to stress. She has just divorced her husband after only 1 year of marriage and is feeling very depressed and stressed about the whole divorce settlement. She has no other health problems and does not take any medications.

Patient History Checklist

☐ Patient's name
☐ Patient's age
☐ Patient's address
☐ Patient's occupation
☐ Patient's presenting complaint
☐ Absence/presence pain
☐ History of the pain
    ☐ Site
    ☐ Onset
    ☐ Duration
    ☐ Intensity
    ☐ Radiation
    ☐ Character
    ☐ Exacerbating factors
    ☐ Relieving factors
    ☐ Medications used to relieve symptoms
☐ Changes in vision

☐ Presence of dizziness
☐ Presence of nausea/vomiting
☐ Presence of fatigue
☐ Presence of irritability
☐ Difficulty concentrating
☐ Difficulty sleeping
☐ Previous episode of symptoms
☐ History of trauma
☐ Medical history
☐ Hospital admissions
☐ Surgical history
☐ Medications
☐ Family history
  ☐ Heart disease
  ☐ Diabetes
  ☐ Thyroid disease
  ☐ Cancer
  ☐ Psychiatric illnesses
  ☐ Others

Physical Examination Checklist

☐ Overall assessment
☐ Vitals
  ☐ Temperature—assess for fever
  ☐ Pulse
  ☐ Blood pressure
  ☐ Respirations
☐ Evaluate mental status
  ☐ Orientation to person, place, and time
  ☐ Level of consciousness
  ☐ Short-term memory
  ☐ Long-term memory
  ☐ Observe the patient's gait and speech
☐ Examine the head
  ☐ Assess for masses, ecchymosis, lacerations, tenderness

☐ Examine the eyes
    ☐ Assess for papilledema
☐ Examine the ears
    ☐ Assess the external ear canal for fluid drainage
    ☐ Assess the tympanic membranes
☐ Assess for cervical rigidity
☐ Brudzinski's sign
☐ Kernig's sign
☐ Examine all cranial nerves (I–XII)
☐ Examine the sensory system
    ☐ Check for pain and crude touch in all parts of the body
    ☐ Romberg's test
    ☐ Proprioception at fingers and toes
    ☐ Vibratory sense
    ☐ Stereognosis
    ☐ Graphesthesia
    ☐ 2-point discrimination
    ☐ Point localization
    ☐ Extinction
☐ Examine the motor system
    ☐ Inspect the motor system for atrophy, fasciculations, and involuntary movements
    ☐ Palpate all limbs for muscle tone
    ☐ Check all major muscle groups for power
    ☐ Check all reflexes
        ☐ Abdominal
        ☐ Plantar
        ☐ Biceps
        ☐ Triceps
        ☐ Brachioradialis
        ☐ Knee
        ☐ Ankle
☐ Examine the cerebellum
    ☐ Ask the patient to walk in a straight line, heel to toe
    ☐ Ask the patient to walk in a straight line on his/her heels
    ☐ Ask the patient to walk in a straight line on his/her toes
    ☐ Ask the patient to perform the finger–nose test

☐ Ask the patient to perform the knee–heel–shin test
☐ Check for dysdiadochokinesia

Differential Diagnosis

1. Trauma
2. Tension headache
3. Cluster headache
4. Subarachnoid aneurysm (rupture)
5. Temporal arteritis

Follow-Up

1. Pain medication
2. Dietary counseling (avoidance of foods and drinks such as alcohol, caffeine, dairy products, chocolate)
3. Computed tomography scan (CT) (if necessary)
4. Lumbar puncture (LP) (if necessary)

PALPITATIONS

A 43-year-old female is seen in the outpatient department. She describes that she has been experiencing a rather strange sensation in her chest. She describes that she occasionally feels her heart "flutter and bump." She has been noticing this sensation for the past 3 months. She denies any associated shortness of breath. She also denies chest pain and diaphoresis associated with the sensation. She has not had a fever and has been feeling well with the exception of these fluttering sensations. She has had no episodes of dizziness. The patient reports that she has approximately 5–10 episodes per day and has noticed that the majority of them seem to occur while she is at work. She lives at home with her husband and their 4 children. She has recently started back into the workforce as a bank teller for the first time in 12 years and admits that she is finding it very stressful to return to work after so many years away from it.

Patient History Checklist

☐ Patient's name
☐ Patient's age
☐ Patient's address
☐ Patient's occupation
☐ Patient's presenting complaint
☐ Frequency of palpitations
☐ Associated symptoms
   ☐ Diaphoresis
   ☐ Shortness of breath
   ☐ Chest pain
   ☐ Dizziness
☐ Diet
☐ Changes in appetite
☐ Presence of weight loss/gain

☐ Previous episodes of palpitations
☐ Use of nicotine
☐ Use of alcohol
☐ Use of caffeine
☐ Use of diet pills
☐ Use of illicit drugs
☐ Frequency and type of exercise
☐ Stress at present
☐ Medical history
☐ Hospital admissions
☐ Surgical history
☐ Medications
☐ Family history
    ☐ Heart disease
    ☐ Thyroid disease
    ☐ Diabetes
    ☐ Cancer
    ☐ Other

Physical Examination Checklist

☐ Overall assessment
☐ Vitals
    ☐ Temperature
    ☐ Pulse—assess for tachycardia
    ☐ Blood pressure—assess for hypertension
    ☐ Respirations
☐ Examine the neck
    ☐ Examine JVP wave pattern
    ☐ Measure the JVP
    ☐ Carotid arteries—assess for bruits
☐ Cardiovascular system
    ☐ Inspect the precordium
        ☐ Shape
        ☐ Scars

☐ Pulses
☐ Apex
☐ Palpate the precordium
  ☐ Tenderness
  ☐ Pulses
  ☐ Apex
  ☐ Thrill
  ☐ Heaves
☐ Percuss the heart borders
☐ Auscultate with the bell
  ☐ Aortic area
  ☐ Pulmonic area
  ☐ Erb's point
  ☐ Tricuspid area
  ☐ Apex (mitral) area
☐ Auscultate with the diaphragm
  ☐ Aortic area
  ☐ Pulmonic area
  ☐ Erb's point
  ☐ Tricuspid area
  ☐ Apex (mitral) area
☐ Auscultate with the bell—patient in left lateral recumbent position
☐ Auscultate with the bell—patient in aortic position

Differential Diagnosis

1. Anxiety
2. Fever
3. Caffeine/nicotine use
4. Hyperthyroidism
5. Anemia
6. Mitral valve prolapse
7. Electrolyte imbalance

Follow-Up

1. Electrocardiogram (ECG)
2. Echocardiogram (EcHO)
3. Complete blood count (CBC)
4. Thyroid stimulating hormone (TSH)
5. Free thyroxine (T_4)/free triiodothyroxine (T_3)
6. Electrolytes

PANCREATITIS

A 55-year-old male is seen in the emergency department. He is complaining of severe abdominal pain which started several hours ago. The pain is located in the middle/left upper abdominal area and radiates to his lower middle back. The patient relates the pain to eating as he had just finished a large meal before the initial onset of the pain. He describes the pain as a twisting, stabbing pain which has been gradually worsening. He reports that he has had several similar episodes in the past; however, this is the most severe the pain has ever been. On a scale of 1–10, with 10 being the most severe pain, the patient reports that the pain is a 9. He has been feeling nauseated since the onset of the pain and has had multiple episodes of vomiting. He denies diarrhea or constipation and states that vomiting seems to make his pain worse. He denies any fevers. When questioned about alcohol consumption the patient is evasive and answers that he occasionally drinks alcohol. Upon further questioning, the patient states that he drinks approximately ¼ of a bottle of rum per day and has been doing so for the past 8 years. He smokes 1 pack of cigarettes per day. He lives with his wife and their 2 teenage daughters. He has no significant medical history.

Patient History Checklist

☐ Patient's name
☐ Patient's age
☐ Patient's address
☐ Patient's occupation
☐ Patient's presenting complaint
☐ Absence/presence of abdominal pain
☐ History of the pain
   ☐ Site
   ☐ Onset
   ☐ Duration
   ☐ Intensity

- ☐ Radiation
- ☐ Character
- ☐ Exacerbating factors
- ☐ Relieving factors
- ☐ Medications used to try to relieve the pain
- ☐ Previous episodes
- ☐ Presence of weight loss/gain
- ☐ Changes in bowel movements
- ☐ Changes in appetite (increased/decreased)
- ☐ Nausea/vomiting
- ☐ Presence of fever
- ☐ Presence of melena
- ☐ Presence of hematemesis
- ☐ Alcohol use (quantity/duration of use)
- ☐ Cigarette use (quantity/duration of use)
- ☐ Medical history
- ☐ Hospital admissions
- ☐ Surgical history
- ☐ Medications
- ☐ Family history
  - ☐ Gastric ulcers
  - ☐ Heart disease
  - ☐ Diabetes
  - ☐ Thyroid disease
  - ☐ Cancer
  - ☐ Others

Physical Examination Checklist

- ☐ Overall assessment
- ☐ Vitals
  - ☐ Temperature—assess for fever
  - ☐ Pulse—assess for tachycardia
  - ☐ Blood pressure—assess for hypotension
  - ☐ Respirations
- ☐ Examine the abdomen

☐ Inspect
☐ Auscultate
☐ Light palpation
☐ Deep palpation
☐ Assess for organomegaly (palpation and percussion)
☐ Assess for muscular rigidity
☐ Assess for rebound tenderness
☐ Indicate to the patient that you would like to perform a digital rectal examination but will not do so during this examination

Differential Diagnosis

1. Cholecystitis
2. Gastroesophageal reflux
3. Alcoholic gastritis
4. Hepatitis
5. Esophageal spasm

Follow-Up

1. Digital rectal examination (DRE)
2. Amylase level
3. Lipase level
4. Stool guiac
5. Complete blood count (CBC)
6. Liver function tests (LFTs)
7. Abdominal ultrasound

PELVIC INFLAMMATORY DISEASE

A 16-year-old female is seen in the emergency department. She has been experiencing severe abdominal pain for the past 24 hours. She has been febrile over the same period of time. The pain is localized to her pelvic region particularly on her right side. She describes the pain as a sharp pain—a 6 on a scale of 1–10 with 10 being the most severe. She has been feeling nauseated over the past 24 hours and has vomited 3 times. Her appetite has been very poor although she has been trying to take sips of fluids since the onset of the symptoms. She has noticed that she has been having some vaginal discharge for the past 2 weeks. The discharge is greenish in color and has a foul odor. She has not experienced any dysuria. She is sexually active with 1 partner and denies ever having any sexually transmitted diseases in the past. She is taking oral contraceptives and admits that she and her partner do not take any precautions against sexually transmitted diseases.

Patient History Checklist

☐ Patient's name
☐ Patient's age
☐ Patient's address
☐ Patient's occupation
☐ Patient's presenting complaint
☐ Sexual history
   ☐ Age of menarche
   ☐ Frequency of periods
   ☐ Last menstrual period
   ☐ Duration of periods
   ☐ Presence of dysmenorrhea
   ☐ Frequency of sexual intercourse
   ☐ Interest in sexual intercourse
   ☐ Method of birth control
   ☐ Use of condoms

- ☐ History of sexually transmitted diseases
- ☐ Presence of vaginal discharge
- ☐ Presence of dyspareunia
- ☐ Number of pregnancies/outcomes of pregnancies
- ☐ Number of abortions
- ☐ Reasons for abortions
- ☐ Presence of weight loss/gain
- ☐ Partner's details
  - ☐ Age
  - ☐ Occupation
  - ☐ History of sexually transmitted diseases
  - ☐ Number of sexual partners
  - ☐ Number of children, if any
- ☐ Medical history
- ☐ Hospital admissions
- ☐ Surgical history
- ☐ Medications
- ☐ Family history
  - ☐ Heart disease
  - ☐ Diabetes
  - ☐ Hypertension
  - ☐ Cancer
  - ☐ Others
- ☐ Social history
  - ☐ Smoking
  - ☐ Alcohol
  - ☐ Other drug use
  - ☐ Family situation

Physical Examination Checklist

- ☐ Overall assessment
- ☐ Vitals
  - ☐ Temperature—assess for fever
  - ☐ Pulse—assess for tachycardia

- ☐ Blood pressure—assess for hypotension
- ☐ Respirations
- ☐ Examine the abdomen
  - ☐ Inspect
  - ☐ Auscultate
  - ☐ Light palpation
  - ☐ Deep palpation
  - ☐ Assess for organomegaly (palpation and percussion)
  - ☐ Assess for muscular rigidity
  - ☐ Assess for rebound tenderness
- ☐ Indicate to the patient that you would like to perform a pelvic examination including vaginal cultures but will not do so during this examination

Differential Diagnosis

1. Bacterial infection
2. Appendicitis
3. Meckel's diverticulitis
4. Ectopic pregnancy

Follow-Up

1. Bimanual pelvic examination
2. Vaginal cultures
3. Complete blood count (CBC)
4. Abdominal ultrasound
5. Beta human chorionic gonadotrophin (β-HCG)

PERIPHERAL VASCULAR DISEASE

A 59-year-old female is seen in the clinic. She has been experiencing pain in her left calf while walking. She has always enjoyed walking. However, since the onset of this pain she has decreased the amount of walking that she has been doing. The pain starts after walking about half a mile and she describes the pain as a dull aching pain. She usually stops for about 5 minutes when she experiences the pain and the pain resolves. However, it comes back again after walking the same distance. Her medical history is significant for hypertension for the past 15 years. She smokes 2 packs of cigarettes a day and has done so for the past 45 years. She denies the use of alcohol.

Patient History Checklist

- ☐ Patient's name
- ☐ Patient's age
- ☐ Patient's address
- ☐ Patient's occupation
- ☐ Patient's presenting complaint
- ☐ Presence of pain
- ☐ History of the pain
  - ☐ Site
  - ☐ Onset
  - ☐ Duration
  - ☐ Intensity
  - ☐ Radiation
  - ☐ Character
  - ☐ Exacerbating factors
  - ☐ Relieving factors
- ☐ History of vascular disease
- ☐ History of diabetes
- ☐ History of hypertension

- ☐ Presence of weight loss/gain
- ☐ Medical history
- ☐ Hospital admissions
- ☐ Surgical history
- ☐ Medications
- ☐ Family history
  - ☐ Heart disease
  - ☐ Diabetes
  - ☐ Hypertension
  - ☐ Cancer
  - ☐ Others
- ☐ Social history
  - ☐ Smoking
  - ☐ Alcohol
  - ☐ Other drug use

Physical Examination Checklist

- ☐ Overall assessment
- ☐ Vitals
  - ☐ Temperature
  - ☐ Pulse
  - ☐ Blood pressure
  - ☐ Respirations
- ☐ Inspect the upper and lower extremities for size and symmetry
- ☐ Examine the nails, hair, and skin
- ☐ Observe any ulcers or gangrene taking care to examine the soles of the feet
- ☐ Palpate temperature in both the upper and the lower extremities comparing both sides
- ☐ Palpate pulses
  - ☐ Dorsalis pedis
  - ☐ Posterior tibial
  - ☐ Popliteal
  - ☐ Femoral

- ☐ Radial
- ☐ Ulnar
- ☐ Brachial
- ☐ Perform Allen's test
- ☐ Perform Buerger's test
- ☐ Check for bruits over the abdominal aorta and both the iliofemoral arteries
- ☐ Examine the motor system
    - ☐ Inspect the motor system for atrophy, fasciculations, and involuntary movements
    - ☐ Palpate all limbs for muscle tone
    - ☐ Check all major muscle groups for power
    - ☐ Check all reflexes
        - ☐ Abdominal
        - ☐ Plantar
        - ☐ Biceps
        - ☐ Triceps
        - ☐ Brachioradialis
        - ☐ Knee
        - ☐ Ankle
- ☐ Examine the sensory system
    - ☐ Check for pain and crude touch in all parts of the body
    - ☐ Romberg's test
    - ☐ Proprioception at fingers and toes
    - ☐ Vibratory sense
    - ☐ Stereognosis
    - ☐ Graphesthesia
    - ☐ 2-point discrimination
    - ☐ Point localization
    - ☐ Extinction
- ☐ If time permits perform a full cardiovascular examination

Differential Diagnosis

1. Trauma
2. Buerger's disease
3. Lumbar disc degeneration
4. Abdominal aneurysm
5. Cardiac disease and systemic embolism

Follow-Up

1. Doppler ultrasound of the lower limb arteries
2. Electrocardiogram (ECG)
3. X-ray of the lumbar spine
4. Lipid profile
5. Fasting blood glucose

PNEUMONIA

A 65-year-old female is admitted to the hospital after being brought to the emergency department by her daughter. She has had a productive cough for the past 3 days. Her sputum is yellow/green. She has also been experiencing some difficulty breathing since the onset of the cough. She has had intermittent chest pain related to the coughing. She has been febrile at home with a temperature ranging from 99–101°F. Her only significant medical history is arthritis which she developed at a young age. She is fairly disabled from this at this point. She has a difficult time getting around and relies on her daughter to help her with most daily activities including dressing and using the toilet. She has had no ill contacts that she is aware of. She has never experienced these symptoms before.

Patient History Checklist

☐ Patient's name
☐ Patient's age
☐ Patient's address
☐ Patient's occupation
☐ Patient's presenting complaint
☐ Duration of symptoms
☐ Presence of cough (productive/nonproductive)
☐ Appearance of the sputum
☐ Presence of blood in the sputum
☐ Shortness of breath
☐ Presence of fever
☐ Presence of rhinorrhea
☐ Presence of chest pain
☐ History of the pain
    ☐ Site
    ☐ Onset
    ☐ Duration

☐ Intensity
☐ Radiation
☐ Character
☐ Exacerbating factors
☐ Relieving factors
☐ Nausea/vomiting
☐ History of weight loss
☐ Presence of night sweats
☐ Ill contacts
☐ Medical history
☐ Hospital admissions
☐ Surgical history
☐ Medications
☐ Family history
   ☐ Cancer
   ☐ Heart disease
   ☐ Diabetes
   ☐ Thyroid disease
   ☐ Asthma/allergies
   ☐ Others
☐ Social history
   ☐ Smoking
   ☐ Alcohol
   ☐ Other drug use

Physical Examination Checklist

☐ Overall assessment
☐ Vitals
   ☐ Temperature—assess for fever
   ☐ Pulse—assess for tachycardia
   ☐ Blood pressure—assess for hypotension
   ☐ Respirations—assess for tachypnea
☐ Examine the face
   ☐ Assess mucous membranes for the presence of cyanosis
☐ Examine the neck

- ☐ Assess for lymphadenopathy
- ☐ Assess for use of accessory muscles
- ☐ Assess the position of the trachea
☐ Examine the extremities
- ☐ Assess for clubbing
- ☐ Assess for cyanosis
☐ Respiratory system — examine the thorax
- ☐ Inspect
  - ☐ Size
  - ☐ Shape
  - ☐ Symmetry
  - ☐ Movement
  - ☐ Deformities of the ribs
  - ☐ Deformities of the spine
  - ☐ Scars
- ☐ Palpate
  - ☐ Tenderness
  - ☐ Excursion
  - ☐ Tactile fremitus
  - ☐ Chest dimensions
  - ☐ Position of the diaphragm
- ☐ Percuss
  - ☐ All areas comparing side to side
  - ☐ Diaphragm excursion (left)
  - ☐ Diaphragm excursion (right)
- ☐ Auscultate
  - ☐ All areas comparing side to side
  - ☐ Breath sounds
  - ☐ Vocal resonance
  - ☐ Whispering pectoriloquy
  - ☐ Aegophony

Differential Diagnosis

1. Tuberculosis
2. Lung abscess
3. Bronchitis
4. Bronchiectasis

Follow-Up

1. Chest x-ray (CXR)
2. Sputum culture
3. Computed tomography scan (CT)
4. Bronchoscopy

PNEUMOTHORAX

A 34-year-old female is seen in the outpatient clinic. She complains of severe left-sided chest pain. She also complains that she is having difficulty breathing. She finds that she is unable to catch her breath. The pain and the shortness of breath came on very suddenly approximately 2 hours prior to her visit to the clinic. The pain is constant and any movement seems to make the pain much worse. She also complains that she has had a cough for the past month following a flu and that every time she coughs or sneezes the pain is much worse. She has not been febrile at home. She denies nausea or vomiting. She feels like her heart is beating much faster than usual. She has never experienced these symptoms in the past. She has had no ill contacts and denies any recent travel out of the country. She lives at home with her husband and their 2 children, all of whom are well. Her medical history is unremarkable. She smokes about 10 cigarettes a day and denies the use of alcohol. She is currently taking an oral contraceptive medication.

Patient History Checklist

- ☐ Patient's name
- ☐ Patient's age
- ☐ Patient's address
- ☐ Patient's occupation
- ☐ Patient's presenting complaint
- ☐ Duration of symptoms
- ☐ Presence of cough (productive/nonproductive)
- ☐ Appearance of the sputum
- ☐ Presence of blood in the sputum
- ☐ Shortness of breath
- ☐ Presence of chest pain
- ☐ Time of onset of shortness of breath/chest pain
- ☐ Presence of fever
- ☐ Presence of diaphoresis

- ☐ Presence of rhinorrhea
- ☐ History of the pain
  - ☐ Site
  - ☐ Onset
  - ☐ Duration
  - ☐ Intensity
  - ☐ Radiation
  - ☐ Character
  - ☐ Exacerbating factors
  - ☐ Relieving factors
- ☐ Nausea/vomiting
- ☐ Recent illnesses
- ☐ History of weight loss
- ☐ Presence of night sweats
- ☐ Pain or swelling of the lower extremities
- ☐ Ill contacts
- ☐ Medical history
- ☐ Hospital admissions
- ☐ Surgical history
- ☐ Medications
- ☐ Family history
  - ☐ Cancer
  - ☐ Heart disease
  - ☐ Diabetes
  - ☐ Thyroid disease
  - ☐ Asthma/allergies
  - ☐ Others
- ☐ Social history
  - ☐ Smoking
  - ☐ Alcohol
  - ☐ Other drug use

Physical Examination Checklist

- ☐ Overall assessment
- ☐ Vitals

☐ Temperature—assess for fever
☐ Pulse—assess for tachycardia
☐ Blood pressure
☐ Respirations—assess for tachypnea
☐ Examine the face
　☐ Assess mucous membranes for the presence of cyanosis
☐ Examine the neck
　☐ Assess for lymphadenopathy
　☐ Assess for use of accessory muscles
　☐ Assess the position of the trachea
☐ Examine the extremities
　☐ Assess for clubbing
　☐ Assess for cyanosis
☐ Respiratory system—examine the thorax
　☐ Inspect
　　☐ Size
　　☐ Shape
　　☐ Symmetry
　　☐ Movement
　　☐ Deformities of the ribs
　　☐ Deformities of the spine
　　☐ Scars
　☐ Palpate
　　☐ Tenderness
　　☐ Excursion
　　☐ Tactile fremitus
　　☐ Chest dimensions
　　☐ Position of the diaphragm
　☐ Percuss
　　☐ All areas comparing side to side
　　☐ Diaphragm excursion (left)
　　☐ Diaphragm excursion (right)
　☐ Auscultate
　　☐ All areas comparing side to side
　　☐ Breath sounds
　　☐ Vocal resonance

☐ Whispering pectoriloquy
☐ Aegophony
☐ Perform a full cardiovascular examination if time permits

Differential Diagnosis

1. Pneumonia
2. Myocardial infarction
3. Pulmonary infarct
4. Lung abscess
5. Bronchitis
6. Congestive heart failure
7. Bronchospasm

Follow-Up

1. Chest x-ray (CXR)
2. Arterial blood gases (ABGs)
3. Oxygen supplementation, as needed
4. Pain medication
5. Chest tube

RHEUMATOID ARTHRITIS

A 32-year-old female is seen by her primary care physician. She complains that she has been having difficulty with her hands and her knees for the past 6 months. She reports that the first time that she experienced the symptoms was in the morning. She states that at the onset of her symptoms she felt very stiff in the mornings for approximately 30 minutes and then the stiffness would resolve and not reappear again until the next morning. She complains that the symptoms have been getting progressively worse over the past 6 months and she is now having difficulty with her normal daily activities. She still experiences a great deal of stiffness in the morning, but now the stiffness does not resolve until after lunch. She also has noticed that she has been feeling stiff in the evenings while watching television. She has been very fatigued over the past 6 months and finds that she is having difficulty doing basic household chores as she now goes to bed just after dinner in the evenings. She has had to miss quite a few days of work due to the severity of her symptoms. She works as a personal secretary and on occasion has had difficulty taking shorthand and typing. She lives alone. She denies the use of cigarettes and alcohol. Her medical history is unremarkable.

Patient History Checklist

☐ Patient's name
☐ Patient's age
☐ Patient's address
☐ Patient's occupation
☐ Patient's presenting complaint
☐ Absence/presence of pain
☐ History of the pain
  ☐ Site
  ☐ Onset
  ☐ Duration
  ☐ Intensity

- ☐ Radiation
- ☐ Character
- ☐ Exacerbating factors
- ☐ Relieving factors
- ☐ Medications used to relieve symptoms
- ☐ Presence of pain on movement
- ☐ Swelling of the affected area
- ☐ Redness of the affected area
- ☐ Presence of Raynaud's phenomenon
- ☐ Presence of nausea/vomiting
- ☐ Presence of fatigue
- ☐ Presence of fever
- ☐ Presence of irritation and/or redness of the eyes
- ☐ Presence of morning stiffness
- ☐ Previous episodes of symptoms
- ☐ History of trauma
- ☐ History of recent surgery
- ☐ Frequency of micturition
- ☐ Presence of dysuria
- ☐ Use of diuretics
- ☐ History of alcoholic binge drinking
- ☐ History of unusual exercise
- ☐ Medical history
- ☐ Hospital admissions
- ☐ Surgical history
- ☐ Medications
- ☐ Family history
  - ☐ Rheumatoid arthritis
  - ☐ Heart disease
  - ☐ Diabetes
  - ☐ Thyroid disease
  - ☐ Cancer
  - ☐ Others
- ☐ Social history
  - ☐ Smoking
  - ☐ Alcohol
  - ☐ Other drug use

Physical Examination Checklist

- ☐ Overall assessment
- ☐ Vitals
  - ☐ Temperature
  - ☐ Pulse
  - ☐ Blood pressure
  - ☐ Respirations
- ☐ Observe patient's gait
- ☐ Examine the extremities (bilaterally)
  - ☐ Inspect upper extremities
    - ☐ Symmetry
    - ☐ Deformities
    - ☐ Swellings
    - ☐ Areas of erythema
  - ☐ Palpate upper extremities
    - ☐ Temperature
    - ☐ Tenderness
    - ☐ Masses
  - ☐ Inspect lower extremities
    - ☐ Symmetry
    - ☐ Deformities
    - ☐ Swellings
    - ☐ Areas of erythema
  - ☐ Palpate lower extremities
    - ☐ Temperature
    - ☐ Tenderness
    - ☐ Masses
- ☐ Assess mobility of hip joints
- ☐ Assess mobility of knee joints
- ☐ Assess mobility of ankle joints
- ☐ Assess mobility of finger joints
- ☐ Assess mobility of foot joints
- ☐ Check all reflexes
  - ☐ Abdominal
  - ☐ Plantar

- ☐ Biceps
- ☐ Triceps
- ☐ Brachioradialis
- ☐ Quadriceps
- ☐ Knee
- ☐ Ankle
- ☐ Examine the eyes, paying particular attention to any inflammation of the conjunctiva or the iris

Differential Diagnosis

1. Osteoarthritis
2. Systemic lupus erythematosus
3. Bursitis
4. Tendonitis
5. Hepatitis

Follow-Up

1. X-rays of affected joints
2. Rheumatoid factor (RF)
3. Erythrocyte sedimentation rate (ESR)
4. Joint aspiration and synovial fluid microscopy
5. Nonsteroidal anti-inflammatory drugs (NSAIDs)
6. Complete blood count (CBC)

SCHIZOPHRENIA

A 22-year-old female is brought to the emergency department by her stepfather who complains of her recent strange behavior. He reports that the patient has been slightly confused lately as well as having episodes of delusions. Upon asking the patient some questions it is discovered that she has been having some paranoid delusions regarding some of the members of the church which she is involved in. She states that the other members of the church whisper behind her back and are plotting against her. She also states that she is quite sure that her mother and her stepfather are also in on the plan and that she cannot trust them to help her. She states that there is nothing wrong with her and feels that her stepfather bringing her to the emergency department is all part of the same sinister plan against her. She goes on to say that these people can't hurt her because she is well protected by Jesus. She states that Jesus has placed a shield around her, protecting her from them. Past history suggests that the patient did not do well in school, had very few friends, and spent most of the time by herself. She smokes approximately 1½ packs of cigarettes per day and admits that she occasionally drinks alcohol, but will not quantify how much or how often she drinks.

Patient History Checklist

- ☐ Patient's name
- ☐ Patient's age
- ☐ Patient's address
- ☐ Patient's occupation
- ☐ Patient's presenting complaint
- ☐ Duration of symptoms
- ☐ Presence of irritability
- ☐ Difficulty concentrating
- ☐ Presence of hallucinations
- ☐ Presence of delusions
- ☐ Presence of disorganized thinking
- ☐ Presence of agitation

- [ ] Lack of initiative
- [ ] Lack of emotional responses
- [ ] Difficulty sleeping
- [ ] Loss of appetite
- [ ] Presence of weight loss/gain
- [ ] Previous episode of symptoms
- [ ] Suicidal ideation
  - [ ] Suicide plan
  - [ ] Previous suicide attempts
- [ ] Homicidal ideation
- [ ] Medical history
- [ ] Hospital admissions
- [ ] Surgical history
- [ ] Medications
- [ ] Family history
  - [ ] Psychiatric illnesses
  - [ ] Depression
  - [ ] Heart disease
  - [ ] Diabetes
  - [ ] Thyroid disease
  - [ ] Cancer
  - [ ] Others
- [ ] Social history
  - [ ] Smoking
  - [ ] Alcohol
  - [ ] Other drug use
  - [ ] Family situation
  - [ ] Work situation
  - [ ] Ability to function at work
  - [ ] Ability to function at home
  - [ ] Presence of support system

Physical Examination Checklist

- [ ] Evaluate mental status
  - [ ] Orientation to person, place, and time

☐ Level of consciousness
☐ Short-term memory
☐ Long-term memory
☐ Abstract or concrete thinking
☐ Mood and affect
☐ Observe the patient's gait and speech
☐ Perform a complete physical examination if time permits

Differential Diagnosis

1. Brief psychotic disorder
2. Drug use
3. Delusional disorder
4. Schizoaffective disorder
5. Schizophreniform disorder
6. Hypothyroidism

Follow-Up

1. Psychiatric evaluation
2. Anti-psychotic medications
3. Blood alcohol level
4. Toxicology (drug screening)
5. Thyroid stimulating hormone (TSH)
6. Free thyroxine (T_4)/free triiodothyroxine (T_3)
7. Counseling

SEVERE ACUTE RESPIRATORY SYNDROME (SARS)

A 49-year-old male is seen complaining of severe shortness of breath. He reports that he first noticed the shortness of breath one day prior, following his return home from a business trip. He also complains of a cough, fever, and occasional diarrhea over the past 24 hours. His maximum temperature at home was 102.5°F. His cough is nonproductive. He complains of feeling muscle aches in his legs and his arms. He has been healthy in the past. He was seen for his annual physical examination one month ago at which time his primary care physician stated that he was in good health. He does not smoke cigarettes and occasionally drinks alcohol. On further questioning about his recent business trip the patient reveals that the business trip had been to China. He denies any knowledge of ill contacts.

Patient History Checklist

☐ Patient's name
☐ Patient's age
☐ Patient's address
☐ Patient's occupation
☐ Patient's presenting complaint
☐ Duration of symptoms
☐ Presence of cough (productive/nonproductive)
☐ Appearance of the sputum
☐ Presence of blood in the sputum
☐ Shortness of breath
☐ Presence of fever
☐ Presence of headache
☐ Presence of malaise
☐ Presence of chills/rigors
☐ Presence of myalgias
☐ Presence of rhinorrhea
☐ Presence of chest pain

- [ ] History of the pain
  - [ ] Site
  - [ ] Onset
  - [ ] Duration
  - [ ] Intensity
  - [ ] Radiation
  - [ ] Character
  - [ ] Exacerbating factors
  - [ ] Relieving factors
- [ ] Presence of nausea/vomiting
- [ ] Presence of diarrhea
- [ ] History of weight loss
- [ ] Presence of night sweats
- [ ] Ill contacts
- [ ] Recent travel; if so, to which area
- [ ] Medical history
- [ ] Hospital admissions
- [ ] Surgical history
- [ ] Medications
- [ ] Family history
  - [ ] Cancer
  - [ ] Heart disease
  - [ ] Diabetes
  - [ ] Thyroid disease
  - [ ] Asthma/allergies
  - [ ] Others
- [ ] Social history
  - [ ] Smoking
  - [ ] Alcohol
  - [ ] Other drug use

Physical Examination Checklist

- [ ] Overall assessment
- [ ] Vitals
  - [ ] Temperature—assess for fever

- ☐ Pulse—assess for tachycardia
- ☐ Blood pressure
- ☐ Respirations—assess for tachypnea
- ☐ Examine the face
  - ☐ Assess mucous membranes for the presence of cyanosis
- ☐ Examine the neck
  - ☐ Assess for lymphadenopathy
  - ☐ Assess for use of accessory muscles
  - ☐ Assess the position of the trachea
- ☐ Examine the extremities
  - ☐ Assess for cyanosis
- ☐ Respiratory system—examine the thorax
  - ☐ Inspect
    - ☐ Size
    - ☐ Shape
    - ☐ Symmetry
    - ☐ Movement
    - ☐ Deformities of the ribs
    - ☐ Deformities of the spine
    - ☐ Scars
  - ☐ Palpate
    - ☐ Tenderness
    - ☐ Excursion
    - ☐ Tactile fremitus
    - ☐ Chest dimensions
    - ☐ Position of the diaphragm
  - ☐ Percuss
    - ☐ All areas comparing side to side
    - ☐ Diaphragm excursion (left)
    - ☐ Diaphragm excursion (right)
  - ☐ Auscultate
    - ☐ All areas comparing side to side
    - ☐ Breath sounds
    - ☐ Vocal resonance
    - ☐ Whispering pectoriloquy
    - ☐ Aegophony

Differential Diagnosis

1. Viral upper respiratory tract infection
2. Pneumonia
3. Lung abscess
4. Bronchitis
5. Tuberculosis

Follow-Up

1. Respiratory isolation
2. Arterial blood gases (ABGs)
3. Chest x-ray (CXR)
4. Sputum culture
5. Pulmonary function tests (PFTs)
6. Complete blood count (CBC)
7. Creatinine phosphokinase level (CK)
8. Liver function tests (LFTs)
9. Computed tomography scan (CT)
10. Bronchoscopy

STABLE ANGINA

A 65-year-old male is seen in the clinic. He reports that he has been having intermittent chest pain over the past 4–6 months. The pain is located on the left side of his chest and occasionally radiates to his left arm. He describes the pain as a squeezing sensation which lasts approximately 25–30 minutes and then subsides. He mainly gets the pain while doing his garden work and denies ever having experienced the pain while at rest. He denies any associated symptoms including shortness of breath, diaphoresis, nausea, or vomiting. He has a medical history significant for hypertension and hypercholesterolemia.

Patient History Checklist

☐ Patient's name
☐ Patient's age
☐ Patient's address
☐ Patient's occupation
☐ Patient's presenting complaint
☐ History of the pain
    ☐ Site
    ☐ Onset
    ☐ Duration
    ☐ Intensity
    ☐ Radiation
    ☐ Character
    ☐ Past experience of this pain
    ☐ Exacerbating factors
    ☐ Relieving factors
    ☐ Medications taken to relieve the pain

☐ Associated factors (sweating, palpitations, shortness of breath, feel-
  ings of anxiety, feeling of impending doom)
☐ Pain in relation to meals
☐ Presence of weight loss/gain
☐ Risk factors
  ☐ Family history
  ☐ Hypertension
  ☐ Diabetes
  ☐ Previous heart condition
  ☐ Smoking
  ☐ Alcohol
  ☐ Exercise
  ☐ Occupation
  ☐ Stress at present
☐ Medical history
☐ Hospital admissions
☐ Surgical history
☐ Medications

Physical Examination Checklist

☐ Overall assessment
☐ Vitals
  ☐ Temperature
  ☐ Pulse—assess for tachycardia
  ☐ Blood pressure—assess for hypertension
  ☐ Respirations
☐ Examine the neck
  ☐ Examine JVP wave pattern
  ☐ Measure the JVP
  ☐ Carotid arteries—assess for upstrokes and the presence of bruits
☐ Cardiovascular system
  ☐ Inspect the precordium
    ☐ Shape
    ☐ Scars

- ☐ Pulses
- ☐ Apex
- ☐ Palpate the precordium
  - ☐ Tenderness
  - ☐ Pulses
  - ☐ Apex
  - ☐ Thrill
  - ☐ Heaves
- ☐ Percuss the heart borders
- ☐ Auscultate with the bell
  - ☐ Aortic area
  - ☐ Pulmonic area
  - ☐ Erb's point
  - ☐ Tricuspid area
  - ☐ Apex (mitral) area
- ☐ Auscultate with the diaphragm
  - ☐ Aortic area
  - ☐ Pulmonic area
  - ☐ Erb's point
  - ☐ Tricuspid area
  - ☐ Apex (mitral) area
- ☐ Auscultate with the bell — patient in left lateral recumbent position
- ☐ Auscultate with the bell — patient in aortic position

Differential Diagnosis

1. Myocardial infarction
2. Pleuritis
3. Pneumonia
4. Musculoskeletal pain
5. Trauma

Follow-Up

1. Electrocardiogram (ECG)
2. Cardiac enzymes (CK, CK-MB, Troponin)
3. Chest x-ray (CXR)
4. Echocardiogram (EcHO)
5. Stress test
6. Lipid profile

TOBACCO CESSATION

A 29-year-old male is seen in the clinic. He is requesting advice on quitting smoking. He has smoked since the age of 15 and smokes 40 cigarettes per day. He has had repeated attempts at quitting with the longest period of abstinence being 3 weeks. He lives at home with his wife, who also smokes. He finds that the fact that his wife also smokes makes it very difficult for him to quit. In the past he has tried nicotine gum and nicotine patches on different occasions. He has never had any medical problems in the past and has never been hospitalized. He does not use alcohol or any illicit drugs.

Patient History Checklist

- [ ] Patient's name
- [ ] Patient's age
- [ ] Patient's address
- [ ] Patient's occupation
- [ ] Patient's presenting complaint
- [ ] Years of cigarette use
- [ ] Number of cigarettes smoked per day
- [ ] Prior attempts at smoking cessation
- [ ] Prior medications/methods used for smoking cessation
- [ ] Partner/friends smoking
- [ ] Presence of productive cough
- [ ] Medical history
- [ ] Hospital admissions
- [ ] Surgical history
- [ ] Medications
- [ ] Family history
  - [ ] Cancer
  - [ ] Heart disease
  - [ ] Diabetes
  - [ ] Thyroid disease

- ☐ Asthma/allergies
- ☐ Others
☐ Social history
- ☐ Alcohol
- ☐ Other drug use

Physical Examination Checklist

☐ If a physical examination is required, perform an assessment of the respiratory system

Follow-Up

1. Nicotine patch/gum
2. Zyban
3. Counseling

TRANSIENT ISCHEMIC ATTACK

A 65-year-old female is brought to the emergency department by her husband. He reports that approximately 4 hours ago he noticed that his wife had developed some difficulty with her speech. She seemed to be confusing object's names. About 1 month ago she had an episode where she complained that she could not open her left eye, but this only lasted a few seconds. She now gives a clear history with normal speech. Her medical history is significant for hypertension and 2 previous heart attacks. She has not experienced chest pain with this episode. She used to smoke cigarettes, about a pack per day, but gave up smoking 3 years ago at the time of her first heart attack. She lives at home with her husband.

Patient History Checklist

- ☐ Patient's name
- ☐ Patient's age
- ☐ Patient's address
- ☐ Patient's occupation
- ☐ Patient's presenting complaint
- ☐ Time of onset of symptoms
- ☐ Previous episode of symptoms
- ☐ Presence of aphasia
- ☐ Presence of ataxia
- ☐ Presence of numbness
- ☐ Presence of loss of motor function
- ☐ Episodes of impaired vision
- ☐ History of abnormal movements and/or tremors
- ☐ Incontinence of urine
- ☐ Presence of dizziness
- ☐ Presence of nausea/vomiting
- ☐ Presence of fatigue

- [ ] Presence of irritability
- [ ] Difficulty concentrating
- [ ] Difficulty sleeping
- [ ] Presence of chest pain
- [ ] Presence of shortness of breath
- [ ] Risk factors
    - [ ] Hypertension
    - [ ] Heart disease
    - [ ] Diabetes mellitus
    - [ ] History of transient ischemic attacks
    - [ ] Cigarette smoking
- [ ] History of trauma
- [ ] Medical history
- [ ] Hospital admissions
- [ ] Surgical history
- [ ] Medications, including over-the-counter medications, prescription medications, and illicit drugs

Physical Examination Checklist

- [ ] Overall assessment
- [ ] Vitals
    - [ ] Temperature
    - [ ] Pulse—assess for arrhythmias
    - [ ] Blood pressure—assess for hypertension
    - [ ] Respirations
- [ ] Evaluate mental status
    - [ ] Orientation to person, place, and time
    - [ ] Level of consciousness
    - [ ] Short-term memory
    - [ ] Long-term memory
    - [ ] Observe the patient's gait and speech
- [ ] Examine the head
    - [ ] Assess for masses, ecchymosis, lacerations, tenderness
    - [ ] Examine the tongue for bite injury

- ☐ Examine the ears
  - ☐ Assess the external ear canal for fluid drainage
  - ☐ Assess the tympanic membranes
- ☐ Examine all cranial nerves (I–XII)
- ☐ Examine the sensory system
  - ☐ Check for pain and crude touch in all parts of the body
  - ☐ Romberg's test
  - ☐ Proprioception at fingers and toes
  - ☐ Vibratory sense
  - ☐ Stereognosis
  - ☐ Graphesthesia
  - ☐ 2-point discrimination
  - ☐ Point localization
  - ☐ Extinction
- ☐ Examine the motor system
  - ☐ Inspect the motor system for atrophy, fasciculations, and involuntary movements
  - ☐ Palpate all limbs for muscle tone
  - ☐ Check all major muscle groups for power
  - ☐ Check all reflexes
    - ☐ Abdominal
    - ☐ Plantar
    - ☐ Biceps
    - ☐ Triceps
    - ☐ Brachioradialis
    - ☐ Knee
    - ☐ Ankle
- ☐ Examine the cerebellum
  - ☐ Ask the patient to walk in a straight line, heel to toe
  - ☐ Ask the patient to walk in a straight line on his/her heels
  - ☐ Ask the patient to walk in a straight line on his/her toes
  - ☐ Ask the patient to perform the finger–nose test
  - ☐ Ask the patient to perform the knee–heel–shin test
  - ☐ Check for dysdiadochokinesia

Differential Diagnosis

1. Cerebral vascular accident
2. Hypoglycemia
3. Central nervous system mass/tumor
4. Cerebral abscess
5. Subdural hematoma
6. Drug use/abuse
7. Seizure disorder

Follow-Up

1. Computed tomography scan (CT)
2. Tissue plasminogen activator (TPA)
3. Heparin/TPA (if appropriate)
4. Electroencephalogram (EEG)
5. Fasting blood glucose
6. Electrocardiogram (ECG)
7. Toxicology (drug screening)

TUBERCULOSIS

A 59-year-old male has been brought to the emergency department by the police after being found unresponsive in the street. Upon arrival, the patient started to regain consciousness and a strong odor of alcohol was detected on his breath. Several hours later the patient is awake, alert, and oriented. When questioned carefully, the patient admits that he drinks a bottle of vodka a day along with several beers. He is currently living in a halfway house which houses 14 other people. He is unemployed. He has not been feeling well for the past 3 months. He has been experiencing intermittent fevers, chills, and a significant amount of weight loss. He reports that he has been experiencing night sweats and often has to get up in the night to dry off. He developed a cough approximately 3–4 months ago which was associated with some chest pain. He has often seen blood in his sputum but has just assumed that this was associated with his cigarette smoking and would resolve if he gave up smoking. He currently smokes 1 pack of cigarettes per day and has done so for the past 35 years.

Patient History Checklist

- ☐ Patient's name
- ☐ Patient's age
- ☐ Patient's address
- ☐ Patient's occupation
- ☐ Patient's presenting complaint
- ☐ Duration of symptoms
- ☐ Presence of cough (productive/nonproductive)
- ☐ Presence of blood in the sputum
- ☐ Shortness of breath
- ☐ Presence of fever
- ☐ History of weight loss
- ☐ Presence of night sweats
- ☐ Presence of chest pain

☐ History of the pain
   ☐ Site
   ☐ Onset
   ☐ Duration
   ☐ Intensity
   ☐ Radiation
   ☐ Character
   ☐ Exacerbating factors
   ☐ Relieving factors
☐ Ill contacts
☐ Nausea/vomiting/diarrhea
☐ Presence of rhinorrhea
☐ History of delirium tremens
☐ Medical history
☐ Hospital admissions
☐ Surgical history
☐ Medications
☐ Family history
   ☐ Cancer
   ☐ Heart disease
   ☐ Diabetes
   ☐ Thyroid disease
   ☐ Asthma/allergies
   ☐ Others
☐ Social history
   ☐ Smoking
   ☐ Alcohol
   ☐ Other drug use
   ☐ Living situation (crowded conditions)

Physical Examination Checklist

☐ Overall assessment
☐ Vitals
   ☐ Temperature—assess for fever
   ☐ Pulse—assess for tachycardia

- [ ] Blood pressure
- [ ] Respirations—assess for tachypnea
- [ ] Examine the face
  - [ ] Assess mucous membranes for the presence of cyanosis
- [ ] Examine the neck
  - [ ] Assess for lymphadenopathy
  - [ ] Assess for use of accessory muscles
  - [ ] Assess the position of the trachea
- [ ] Examine the extremities
  - [ ] Assess for clubbing
  - [ ] Assess for cyanosis
- [ ] Respiratory system—examine the thorax
  - [ ] Inspect
    - [ ] Size
    - [ ] Shape
    - [ ] Symmetry
    - [ ] Movement
    - [ ] Deformities of the ribs
    - [ ] Deformities of the spine
    - [ ] Scars
  - [ ] Palpate
    - [ ] Tenderness
    - [ ] Excursion
    - [ ] Tactile fremitus
    - [ ] Chest dimensions
    - [ ] Position of the diaphragm
  - [ ] Percuss
    - [ ] All areas comparing side to side
    - [ ] Diaphragm excursion (left)
    - [ ] Diaphragm excursion (right)
  - [ ] Auscultate
    - [ ] All areas comparing side to side
    - [ ] Breath sounds
    - [ ] Vocal resonance
    - [ ] Whispering pectoriloquy
    - [ ] Aegophony

☐ Examine the abdomen
  ☐ General examination for signs of hepatic failure
  ☐ Inspect
  ☐ Auscultate
  ☐ Light palpation
  ☐ Deep palpation
  ☐ Assess for organomegaly (palpation and percussion)
  ☐ Assess for fluid wave
  ☐ Assess for shifting dullness

Differential Diagnosis

1. Pneumonia
2. Lung abscess
3. Bronchitis
4. Aspiration of gastric contents

Follow-Up

1. Respiratory isolation
2. Tuberculin skin test (PPD)
3. Chest x-ray (CXR)
4. Sputum culture
5. Computed tomography scan (CT)
6. Bronchoscopy
7. Alcohol withdrawal precautions
8. Alcohol counseling

UNSTABLE ANGINA

A 69-year-old male is seen in the emergency department complaining of chest pain. The pain is located on the left side of his chest and he describes it as a sharp pain which lasts 30–40 minutes and then subsides. He has been awakened 3 times in the past week because of the pain. He reports that he first experienced the pain approximately 6 months ago. However, at that time he was only experiencing the pain once in a while and usually while doing his gardening. His medical history is only significant for hypertension, which was first diagnosed 25 years ago. He smokes half a pack of cigarettes per day and has done so for the past 45 years. Both his father and two of his brothers died from heart disease. There is no other significant family history.

Patient History Checklist

- ☐ Patient's name
- ☐ Patient's age
- ☐ Patient's address
- ☐ Patient's occupation
- ☐ Patient's presenting complaint
- ☐ History of the pain
  - ☐ Site
  - ☐ Onset
  - ☐ Duration
  - ☐ Intensity
  - ☐ Radiation
  - ☐ Character
  - ☐ Past experience of this pain
  - ☐ Exacerbating factors
  - ☐ Relieving factors
  - ☐ Medications taken to relieve the pain

- [ ] Associated factors (sweating, palpitations, shortness of breath, feelings of anxiety, feeling of impending doom)
- [ ] Pain in relation to meals
- [ ] Presence of weight loss/gain
- [ ] Risk factors
  - [ ] Family history
  - [ ] Hypertension
  - [ ] Diabetes
  - [ ] Previous heart condition
  - [ ] Smoking
  - [ ] Alcohol
  - [ ] Exercise
  - [ ] Occupation
  - [ ] Stress at present
- [ ] Medical history
- [ ] Hospital admissions
- [ ] Surgical history
- [ ] Medications

Physical Examination Checklist

- [ ] Overall assessment
- [ ] Vitals
  - [ ] Temperature
  - [ ] Pulse—assess for tachycardia
  - [ ] Blood pressure—assess for hypertension
  - [ ] Respirations
- [ ] Examine the neck
  - [ ] Examine JVP wave pattern
  - [ ] Measure the JVP
  - [ ] Carotid arteries—assess for bruits
- [ ] Cardiovascular system
  - [ ] Inspect the precordium
    - [ ] Shape
    - [ ] Scars

- [ ] Pulses
- [ ] Apex
- [ ] Palpate the precordium
  - [ ] Tenderness
  - [ ] Pulses
  - [ ] Apex
  - [ ] Thrill
  - [ ] Heaves
- [ ] Percuss the heart borders
- [ ] Auscultate with the bell
  - [ ] Aortic area
  - [ ] Pulmonic area
  - [ ] Erb's point
  - [ ] Tricuspid area
  - [ ] Apex (mitral) area
- [ ] Auscultate with the diaphragm
  - [ ] Aortic area
  - [ ] Pulmonic area
  - [ ] Erb's point
  - [ ] Tricuspid area
  - [ ] Apex (mitral) area
- [ ] Auscultate with the bell—patient in left lateral recumbent position
- [ ] Auscultate with the bell—patient in aortic position
- [ ] A full examination of the respiratory system should be performed, if time permits

Differential Diagnosis

1. Myocardial infarction
2. Coronary artery spasm
3. Pleuritis
4. Pneumonia
5. Musculoskeletal pain
6. Trauma

Follow-Up

1. Electrocardiogram (ECG)
2. Cardiac enzymes (CK, CK-MB, Troponin)
3. Chest x-ray (CXR)
4. Echocardiogram (EcHO)
5. Stress test
6. Lipid profile
7. Counseling for smoking cessation

URINARY TRACT INFECTION

A 19-year-old female complains of severe pain in her abdomen which started 1 day ago. She has also been having some discomfort in her pelvis. She describes the pain as a burning pain which moves along her right side to her back. She states that she has been having some difficulty urinating. She finds that she is going to the bathroom frequently, but is only able to pass small amounts of urine. She has noticed that when she does pass urine she feels a burning sensation. The color of her urine is darker that normal, has a foul odor, and at times has some dark red blood in it. She has never experienced these symptoms before. She denies nausea, vomiting, and fever. She has been very healthy in the past. She denies vaginal discharge although does admit that she is sexually active with multiple partners. She has had no pregnancies. Her family history is unremarkable. She smokes approximately half a pack of cigarettes per day and denies the use of alcohol.

Patient History Checklist

- [ ] Patient's name
- [ ] Patient's age
- [ ] Patient's address
- [ ] Patient's occupation
- [ ] Patient's presenting complaint
- [ ] Absence/presence of abdominal pain
- [ ] History of the pain
  - [ ] Site
  - [ ] Onset
  - [ ] Duration
  - [ ] Intensity
  - [ ] Radiation
  - [ ] Character
  - [ ] Exacerbating factors
  - [ ] Relieving factors

- ☐ Changes in bowel movements
- ☐ Changes in appetite (increased/decreased)
- ☐ Changes in menstrual cycle
- ☐ Frequency of micturition
- ☐ Presence of dysuria
- ☐ Presence of nocturia
- ☐ Presence of hematuria
- ☐ Previous episodes of similar symptoms
- ☐ Presence of vaginal discharge
- ☐ Sexual history
  - ☐ Age of menarche
  - ☐ Frequency of periods
  - ☐ Last menstrual period
  - ☐ Duration of periods
  - ☐ Presence of dysmenorrhea
  - ☐ Age of menopause (if relevant)
  - ☐ Sexual activity
  - ☐ History of sexually transmitted diseases
  - ☐ Practice of safe sex
  - ☐ Number of pregnancies/outcomes of pregnancies
- ☐ Medical history
- ☐ Hospital admissions
- ☐ Surgical history
- ☐ Medications
- ☐ Family history
  - ☐ Kidney disease
  - ☐ Heart disease
  - ☐ Diabetes
  - ☐ Thyroid disease
  - ☐ Cancer
  - ☐ Others
- ☐ Social history
  - ☐ Smoking
  - ☐ Alcohol
  - ☐ Other drug use

Physical Examination Checklist

☐ Overall assessment
☐ Vitals
  ☐ Temperature—assess for fever
  ☐ Pulse—assess for tachycardia
  ☐ Blood pressure
  ☐ Respirations
☐ Examine the abdomen
  ☐ Inspect
  ☐ Auscultate
  ☐ Light palpation
  ☐ Deep palpation
  ☐ Assess for organomegaly (palpation and percussion)
  ☐ Assess for muscular rigidity
  ☐ Assess for rebound tenderness
  ☐ Rovsing's sign
  ☐ Assess for referred rebound tenderness
  ☐ Psoas sign
  ☐ Obturator sign
  ☐ Cutaneous hyperesthesia
☐ Indicate to the patient that you would like to perform a pelvic examination, including vaginal cultures, but will not do so during this examination

Differential Diagnosis

1. Pyelonephritis
2. Vaginitis
3. Pelvic inflammatory disease
4. Appendicitis
5. Herpes simplex type 2

Follow-Up

1. Urinalysis (U/A)
2. Urine culture
3. Bimanual pelvic examination
4. Vaginal examination/vaginal cultures
5. Complete blood count (CBC)